On The Banks of
Holliday Creek

On The Banks of Holliday Creek

David Wright

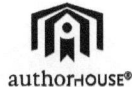

authorHOUSE®

AuthorHouse™
1663 Liberty Drive
Bloomington, IN 47403
www.authorhouse.com
Phone: 1-800-839-8640

Published by AuthorHouse   07/17/2012

ISBN: 978-1-4772-4023-6 (sc)
ISBN: 978-1-4772-4022-9 (hc)
ISBN: 978-1-4772-4024-3 (e)

Library of Congress Control Number: 2012912277

Trailer

After a tragic accident the Wrights find a new beginning moving from the city with all its conveniences to a forty acre farm on the banks of Holliday Creek. Told from the perspective of their nine-year-old son David, the Wrights meet the neighboring Jones family. Dick Wright is a rising star in the Fort Dodge public school system. Old Jim Jones introduces himself as "a flunky who works for United States Gypsum." The two families send their children to Holliday Creek School two miles away. The one-room school thrives under the leadership of Miss Jordison, the teacher you always wished you had. "Each One Teach One" is her process as recalled by the author, David Wright, himself a published educator. Vivid family contrasts are woven into this narrative that shows America in the Truman Era witnessing the advent of electricity, the telephone, and the Baby Boom generation. This book depicts Progressive Republicans confronting forces of social change, Big Government, and Reaction. Underlying this story are the ideals of personal liberty and the challenges of living close to nature.

Contents

Preface

This book is mostly factual, but I have not done tedious historical research. I am a history teacher not a historian, and the one room school house needed to be described by someone who actually attended one. Events are not chronological, but roughly seasonal. The first chapters have a late summer setting. The last chapter happens in the spring. The years are from September 1947 through May 1951.

I have taken liberties in this book; a memoir fictionalized in many parts. It is a little allegorical and you will see the parallel to Adam and Eve in my last chapter *Confligration*. I hope that I have kept characterizations intact. This is a story of two contrasting families who were good neighbors in a rural setting near Fort Dodge, Iowa between 1947 and 1951. Coalville is a real town. Holliday Creek School was a real school. Jack Gorelle and Oren Gray were real people as were all the others I mention. Oren Gray is omniscient. "He could see you from far away." He is "as old as the hills, or eternal." Jack Gorelle does not have these qualities.

During the final phases of my writing, my brother-in law Max Koeper got a phone call from Catherine Ozment, whom he had known as Cathy (Catherine) Jones. In the book she is referred to as Kate. Incredibly, Catherine was trying to contact Fort Dodge people for a get-together. She asked Max if he knew anything of my whereabouts. Max said, "As a matter of fact he is sitting about two feet away from me." He handed me the phone. It was an astounding coincidence.

I met with Catherine, along with Ray Sharf, the husband of another "Jones sister" named Joan. I was saddened to hear that Joan passed away in 2005 after battling cancer for many years. The Jones brothers, Jimmy and Dick, are both gone. Janette passed away in 2005. Catherine made many invaluable contributions to this book. Her memory is sharp and she helped me recall their father, Jim Jones, who was one of the most colorful, genuine people I ever met. Also, I recall the archetypal earth mother Maudie Jones. This book does not intend to judge, but to portray.

You will notice my habit of flipping from the first person in one chapter to the third person in the next. You will also notice that I have been deeply influenced by the poetry of Robert Frost. The chapter "Drawing Water" is like his poem "The Pasture"; "Riding Willows" remembers "Birches," and I quote from his poem "The Line Gang." I was also inspired by Laura Ingalls Wilder, whose novels were read aloud at Holliday Creek School. I would read them to my daughters at bedtime. The title of one of those books, *On the Banks of Plum Creek,* gives rise to the title of this book, *On the Banks of Holliday Creek.* Also, I quote from two poems of Steven Vincent Benét: "The Ballad of William Sycamore" and "The Mountain Whippoorwill." Also, I recall *East of Eden* by John Steinbeck.

My friend, fellow teacher, and football coach, David Archibald, wrote and published an account of his life with his family in Arizona. He challenged me to write of my own boyhood. I took him seriously and I began writing about a year ago. I thank Dave very much.

I invite you into a world I remember.

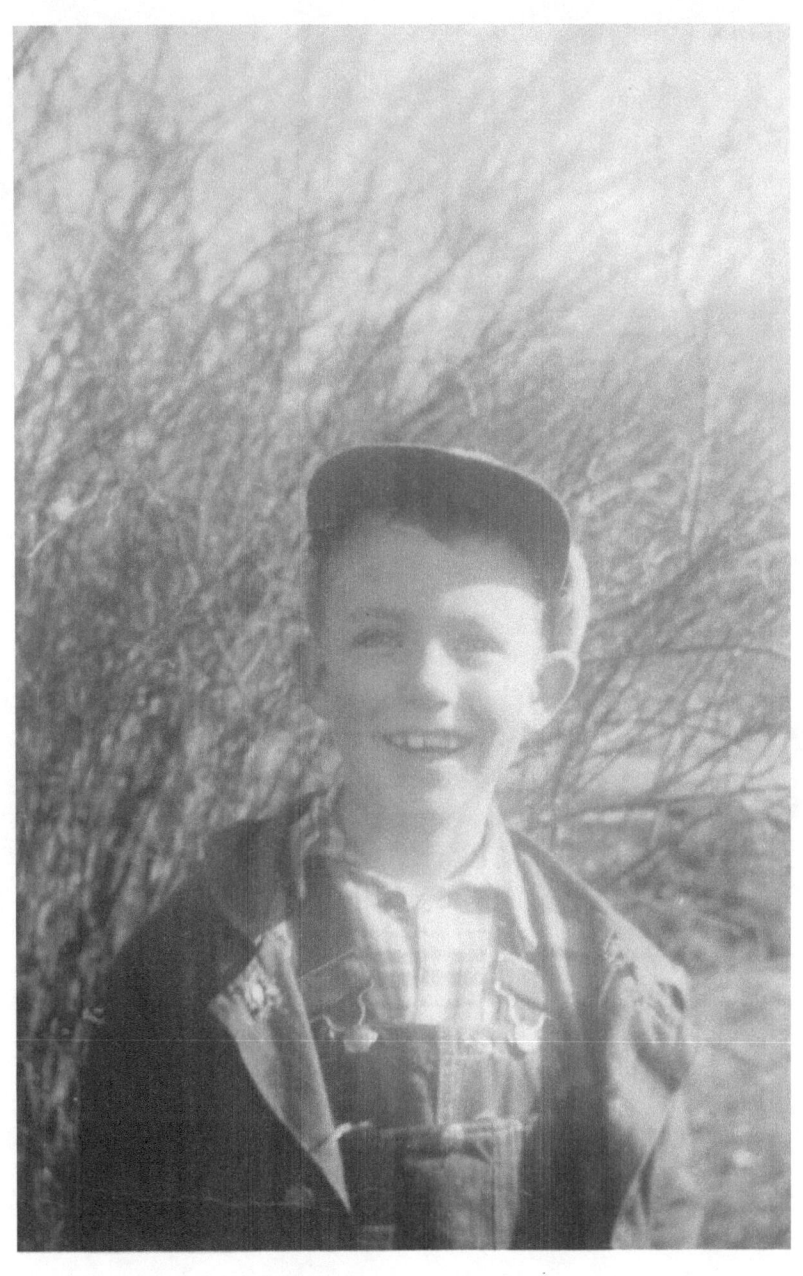

David I. Wright
February 14, 2012

The Class of 1947

The bell rang and I said, "Today is September 5, 2007. This is a new 11th Grade American History class and you all know I'm Dave Wright. Most of you know I have taught here at Academy With Community Partners since I retired from Coronado High in Scottsdale in 2001. I do not need the money but I need to teach. Michael Jordan needed to play basketball long after he had enough money. He still had something big to contribute to the game. I feel the same way, so I pledge to you that I will give you my best game every day. I hope you give me your own best game. I have had many of you in other classes and it is good to see you back. If this is your first trip with me, I say welcome. I am a teacher you will like and trust. Just ask around."

I glanced over in the corner at Kirk, age 18, who I had named ACP's Student of the Block in the spring. He was an ex-gang banger who was back in school studying to become a police officer. He thrived on encouragement and ultra sweet coffee. He waved two fingers at me from behind his Styrofoam cup. He was my Enforcer. Next to him was Kelsie, who was set up for a drug deal and now was on probation. She was back. I had her in class last block. Kelsie would respond to a kind word, and she would confide in me. Next to them was Kevin, a Native American who belonged to a group of hoop dancers and musicians. They had toured Europe, but the trip was over, and he had nowhere to go, so he had come back to finish school. He was passionate about hoop dancing and we would talk about Europe. Over there was Ryan, who had a case pending for his role in a drive-by shooting. He was slick. Next to him Nick was sleeping, but soon he would be flying around the room because he was A.D.H.D. There were new students, and I had already memorized their names. I would get to know them soon. These were my lambs, and I smiled inwardly, remembering the lambs on my family's farm long ago.

I continued. "Right now, over at Sandra Day O'Connor School nearby, we have a kindergarten class getting started. How many kids are in that class?" I asked.

Nick sat up and rubbed his eyes. He had been listening all along. He sometimes would try to get off on a good start at the beginning of a Block. He answered. "They probably have about twenty-five kids in that class, Mr. Wright." He yawned and stretched.

"Right, Nick." I said. "Take your hat off in class, please. How many of them will graduate from high school?"

The kids looked at one another. Nick took his hat off, but he put his head back down.

"Out of a beginning class of twenty-five kindergarteners starting school on September 5, 2007, how many will graduate from high school?" I asked, probing a little deeper, insisting on an answer.

Kirk smiled his half-smirk smile. "Probably two or three of them won't live that long." He took a drink of coffee. I provide coffee and creamer in my class. Kirk gets to class early to get the coffee. He uses too much creamer and sugar. Today there was no jerky, but only apple slices.

What do you mean by that?" I asked.

"Some of them will die before they reach graduation."

"Or go to prison," said Nick, sitting back up.

There was general agreement.

"So," I said, "Maybe twenty or twenty-one will live to be age eighteen and all of those will graduate. Your expectation is that only twenty kids out of that group of twenty-five kindergarteners will ever graduate," I said. "That is 80 percent. Actual statistics show that about 90 percent will graduate, so your expectation is a little low. This reminds me to say that if you guys come to this class every day and give me your best you will have a 90 percent chance of getting credit. What expectation was there for a class of kindergarteners sixty years ago? That would be in 1947."

I leaned back against the white board and took a deep breath. *I had planned this moment for a long time. Now I was going to go through with it.* I was a tough old bird teaching in a charter school called Academy with Community Partners. I started teaching there six weeks after conventional retirement from Scottsdale Coronado High; I was starting my seventh year at ACP. I decided I still loved teaching kids, and retirement bored me. My kids would feed from me, so I went on.

"What expectation was there for a class of kindergarteners sixty years ago? Did you know I started kindergarten sixty years ago today? That was September 5, 1947. That is why I asked the question. There were five of us in my kindergarten class. Back then they did not call it kindergarten, but Primary. I attended a one-room country school in Iowa and I would like to tell you about it during the Block. I graduated from high school in 1960 and Larry Jordison graduated too. He started kindergarten with me in 1947. Two of us out of five graduated. That was only 40 percent of us."

3

When I said I went to a country school, the kids looked at one another, and eyes started to roll back in their heads. They had heard things before from other teachers about walking two miles through the snow each way and having no TV. I knew what I was up against. "I'm a living fossil," I continued. "I'm really some kind of creature out of the past. I never belonged in your world. What happened to those kids who started Primary sixty years ago? I was one of them. I have been told that only about 40 percent of the kids who started school that same day as me ever finished high school, so Larry Jordison and I were about typical. That is the era we will be studying during this Block. It is called the Post War Era and it dates from 1945 to the present." I paused. "Kelsie, when did your mom graduate from high school?"

"She didn't graduate," Kelsie replied. "She was in jail when she should have graduated."

"I did not know that," I said. "I'm sorry to hear about your mother. Do you know when that was?"

She thought a few seconds. I waited for her response. "It would have been in 1977. My brother was born that year. He's thirty. He's in prison again. Mom had me in 1991. She was not in prison when she had me."

"You have a good mind for remembering dates, Kelsie," I said. "That is what I'm trying to say in a book I am writing: You need to remember who you are and what you went through.

"Your brother was part of the Post War Baby Boom. That is the era right at the end of World War II when the returning soldiers made lots of babies. Was your grandfather in World War II?"

"I never met my grandfather, Mr. Wright. Or my dad. You are the only grandfather I ever had."

I did not know what to say to her. I took another deep breath. I loved the kids, but this was to be my last year at ACP. I had been teaching since 1966, but the pain in my spine was unbearable and I did not know how to deal with it. I couldn't actually pour out my life in front of the class. I couldn't last. I was used up, as Saint Paul said it. But if I could have poured it all out, this is what I would have said.

It's Off to School We Go

David knew it was going to be hot at Holliday Creek School, but at seven in the morning, dew was still on the grass. A big grasshopper leaped from a brown grass straw beside David's foot and flew across the road. He wanted to chase after it. It would be a perfect bait to catch a big chub in the Creek beyond the willows. For now, however, he would stand here in his new blue bib overalls, waiting to start the daily walk to school. He glanced over at his mom, who was holding the hand of his four-year-old brother, Johnny. She was looking down the lane. The Jones girls were overdue.

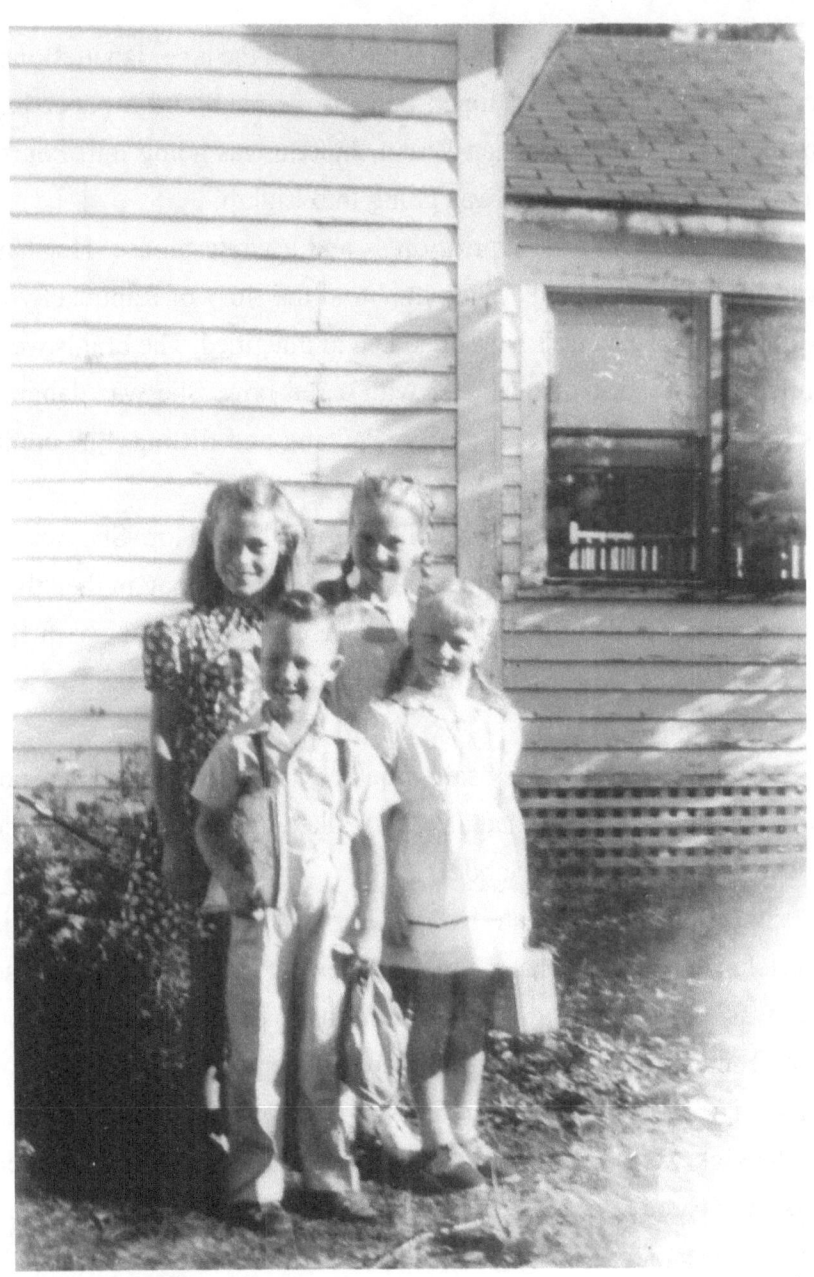

The First Day of School September 1947

They soon appeared, rounding the bend in the lane, Janette Jones leading, carrying a black lunch pail in one hand and a paper bag in another. A year older than David, Janette was going into Fourth grade. Kate followed. She was going into Eighth.

Janette had on a new print dress and a white blouse. Her hair was golden and braided. When they told the story of Rapunzel you would think of Janette's hair, or so David imagined. The braids were coiled on the back of her head with a red bow. She was dancing as she walked. Janette was always dancing and flirting. She could outrun every kid at school except Larry Jordison.

Her older sister Kate wore a blue skirt with a red top. She carried a black lunch pail in one hand and clenched a paper bag in the other. She carried a purse under her arm. There was no red bow in her hair. She walked with deliberateness, but if you played tag she was elusive as quicksilver.

"Hi, Mrs. Wright," they said together. Their sister, Joan was not with them this year. She had already walked up the lane to catch the bus to Fort Dodge High School.

Since Janette and Kate had now arrived, David picked up his black lunch pail in one hand and the paper bag in the other. Inside the bag was a new box of crayons, a handful of pencils, an eraser (left over from last year), a jar of glue with a rubber nipple, and a tablet of paper. The tablet had a picture of Roy Rogers. Down at the bottom of the sack were a six-inch wooden ruler and a pair of blunt-ended scissors. There was also a coloring book with Hopalong Cassidy on the cover. The coloring book depicted cowboy situations. These were the items the letter from the school required him to bring.

He hoped Janette would notice his recently bought bib overalls with a red and white striped polo shirt, and new shoes. The shoes felt stiff and unnatural. He did not wear shoes much in the summertime. He wanted her to notice he had a pencil sticking out of the pocket on the bib. He could have shown her he had his three-blade jackknife in his pocket along with his lucky rabbit's foot. In his hip pocket he had a billfold from his birthday last year. He even had a whole dollar bill in it—a birthday gift from Granddad Bryan, and forty-three cents in the wallet's coin purse to buy pop and ice cream. He carried the billfold even though he would not be anywhere near a store for the rest of the week. His identification said he was David Wright from Rural Route 2, Coalville, Iowa. Date of Birth was May 28, 1942. His weight was listed as seventy-five pounds; his hair, brown; eyes, blue; standing four feet five inches tall. His parents were John Richard Wright and Shirley Wright. The space beside "Telephone" was marked N/P—no telephone. The information was far out of date. He was bigger now. And they had a telephone, along with electricity.

Janette did not notice anything about David.

David's Mom came over to him and hugged him. She did not kiss him because he would be embarrassed. Looking at the three of them, she said, "Do well in school. Make us proud of you. Watch for cars." She did not say, "Do *good* in school." She had taught him the difference.

"We will," they said, and they started to walk.

Johnny ran after David and grabbed the suspenders of his new blue bib overalls.

"Deedee" he cried. "Where are you going, Deedee?"

David turned around and looked at his brother and smiled. "I'm going to school. You can come next year when you are five, but we can play in the hills when I get home this afternoon." Johnny gave David a hug and that was that.

David and the two girls walked up the lane. As they neared the first bend, David looked back and saw his mom watching them as they were about to go out of sight. She waved.

*   *   *

She had brought out a handkerchief from her apron pocket and wiped her eyes. Then she blew her nose because David was going off to school and she thought, "God, take care of David because you didn't take of Richard." *Stop!* she said in her mind, and took Johnny by the hand. This happened every year.

In a flash she relived the circumstances that brought them to Holliday Creek. An old man ran over Richard as he was crossing the street on the way home for lunch. He died an hour later in Mercy Hospital amid screaming, prayers, and cursing. Then there was the funeral, and later David searched under the bed and all through the house for Richard; she remembered telling David that Richard is in Heaven. They cried. She closed her nursery school and they sold the house and moved to the apartment. Dick stayed up nights smoking and blaming himself. She remembered her withdrawal into depression with headaches and that David often slipped out of the apartment and hid. She was not up to chasing him because she was pregnant again, so Dick suggested they buy a farm. They had lived on an uncle's acreage before, during the war when the draft was getting close. You could avoid the draft if you could prove you were a farmer. That farm they nicknamed "The Rat Roost." Dick hated the place, but he was willing to move back to an acreage if he could continue teaching in Fort Dodge. They found a small farm where they could recover. The valley along Holliday Creek promised healing and no busy streets, so they remodeled the house and agreed Dick would commute to his teaching job in town. They did not need income from the farm, but it was a possibility.

*　　*　　*

David waved back at his mom. She did not continue waving; it looked like she was blowing her nose just then and she took Johnny by the hand and walked away. David turned around and resumed his trek. It was two miles away—not much of a walk. He had played running ragged through the hills all summer barefoot. Farm kids did not wear shoes in the summer. Today he had new shoes on and they felt stiff and awkward. He was going to school.

They were going due north, walking above the Creek. David looked below the road to his right. That was east. The Creek was a good quarter of a mile away and forty feet lower in elevation. We paused here and looked because you could see most of the valley with the creek running through it. North from the bridge was mostly pasture, and when the wind blew the grass flat it would shine. The hillsides were dark green with August foliage and crows cawed. It was well known this was a favorite parking spot for lovers from Fort Dodge. They would leave cigarette butts and debris strewn about. The view was spoiled because people also used the lovely spot to dump trash. Fresh cans lay on top of rusted ones along with rotted rags and magazines. The sight made David angry. It is hard to keep a lovely thing. Yet, he looked east over the valley across the Creek, and he could see Oren Gray's new barn below. They had nailed down the galvanized roofing and it reflected the early sun. They walked on, and David looked uphill to the left above the road. Up toward the top of the hill of the hill he knew was the Shack. *Stay away from the shack,* his conscience said.

David wanted to make his parents proud of him. He thought about this a lot. Right now, he was thinking about it because Kate and Janette were going on and on about who was smartest, fastest, and prettiest in the school. They named who was the handsomest boy, the bravest, the strongest, the best speller, the best at marbles shooter and jacks player. Who was best at hop scotch, and the kid with the best penmanship and the best singer? They named many categories and then argued about who was first and second place. They did not mention him even once, and he became jealous.

David could take it no more, and he burst ahead and ran up the road to where a Boxelder tree grew. He set his lunch box down by the road and set the bag of supplies beside it. He broke some branches from the tree and stood in front of the Jones girls holding the leafy branches above his head. "I am going to be the outstanding student this year," he cried, smashing the branches on the road for emphasis. "Outstanding student and King of the Cowboys. The King. I am not doing any more smoking, either," he said. "You hear that?" he yelled, dramatically.

"Roy Rogers is the king of the cowboys," said Janette, mockingly. "Everybody knows that."

"You're too big for your britches," Kate said, walking by him. "Besides, you smoke every chance you get."

"You'll see," David said. "You'll all see." He tossed the branches beside the ditch and picked up the lunch box and paper bag. He hurried to catch up. He was sweating and he could feel the sweat trickle down his back. Sweat mixed with rose-scented hair oil ran down from his scalp to his face.

Soon they were at the corner where the lane met the main road. If you turned right and went east you were headed toward Holliday Creek School a mile and a half away. If you turned left and went up the hill west toward Fort Dodge you would pass by Bob Jordison's place. Using that route you would reach Coalville about a mile and a half beyond. Fort Dodge was another five miles beyond that. David noticed there was a fresh layer of gravel, so there would be less dust than usual when a car drove by. They turned east and the road ran downhill to the bridge. There was a grove of sumac growing at the corner with leaves beginning to turn red along the edges. The leaves were dusty from the gravel road. Small birds pecked at its ripening seeds. There were lots of Black Eyed Susans, goldenrod, and ragweed. They did not give him hay fever. Other people talked about hay fever a lot in September. Weeds were pungent, he thought. He liked that word. Soon they reached the bridge. The Creek ran below. It was a concrete and steel bridge with no superstructure. There were pilings near it where an older bridge once stood.

At the bridge, David stood next to Janette and they looked down into the water sparkling in the sun. The Creek was low because it had not rained. David kicked gravel over the side of the bridge. He loved the splashing sound. Startled pigeons flew out from under the bridge.

"Hush. The trolls will hear you," Janette said, almost whispering. Janette said she believed in trolls. She also said she believed in witches and goblins. David would pretend to believe in them too. It made the Hills kind of scary.

"Up the airy mountain, down the rushy glen; We dare not go a hunting for fear of little men," whispered Janette.

David replied in a whisper. "Wee folk, good folk trooping all together; Green jacket, red cap, and white owl's feather." They had memorized part of the poem from the poetry book that David's mom read to them.

They crossed the bridge and marched off eastward, pretending, and hurried to catch up with Kate. They looked over to Oren Gray's place. Men were at work building the new barn. He raised horses. Oren Gray was a kind old man—as old as the hills, people said. He now stood near his new barn. He waved his straw hat. They waved back. "Have a good year," he shouted. Kate waved again. He did not like kids bothering his horses, but sometimes he would let you ride behind the saddle when he saw you in the hills. He was stooped and walked around his corral with a long walking stick. He was too tall to be a troll, David thought.

Right away they arrived at the Benson's lane across the road and to the north of Oren Gray's. Walter, or "Walt," was running to catch up with his sister Francis. Walt was in First and Francis was in Fourth with Janette. Both Walt and Francis had black lunch pails. And they were both fat. Walt's nose was running as usual. He licked it. He had hay fever.

Unlike the rest of us, the Benson kids didn't have any paper sack of supplies between them.

"Didn't you bring your pencils and paper and stuff?" Kate asked.

"We didn't buy any, so there," Francis said. Walt did not say anything. The Bensons were poor farmers. Cliff Benson sometimes worked for Oren Gray.

The group of five began the steep, long climb up the eastern slope of the valley.

"I suppose you are going to borrow paper and pencils from us like you did all last year," Kate said. Francis did not say anything. Nobody said much on the way up the hill. You saved your breath on the way uphill. Francis said that they were walking too fast. Janette stuck out her tongue, turned around and wiggled her bottom at them and dashed ahead.

At the top of the hill they met the four Sadler kids coming down the lane from their farm. Marlene was in the lead and she walked alone. She had a scowl on her face. Marlene was starting Seventh, and she did not like Kate. Behind them was Betty, who was in Sixth. Betty was always smiling, and she was very kind. She held the hand of Dolores, her little sister who was in First. Roger came dragging behind.

Roger was in Third like David. He was always sad, but today he was wearing a holster with a cap gun.

All the Sadler kids had lunch pails, and each had the mandatory paper bag of supplies.

When Roger saw David, he put down his lunch pail and went for his gun. He pulled the trigger and fired off six real caps at David. Usually boys fanned an imaginary hammer shouting, "Bam-Bam-Bam," but Roger had real caps this time, and they rolled out on top of the gun in a red ribbon, still smoking. David was quick to adapt a cowboy role, and clutched his chest like a man shot. He did not have a gun and holster, along with him because they were against the rules. Everyone knew that, including Roger. David realized this even as he swirled to his left, and in slow motion, fell dead. He lay on the ground and made his left foot twitch twice. It was a good effect. He had done it before. Roger blew not-so-imaginary smoke from his six shooter. Roger was smiling. David was glad he got Roger to smile.

"Get up, David. You're getting all dirty," said Janette. "You show-off."

David got up and dusted off his new bib overalls. His performance was over for now.

"You can't bring cap guns to school," Kate said to Roger.

"Says who?" Marlene Sadler asked. She knew the rules as well as anyone.

"It's a rule," said Kate.

We all looked at one another. Would they fight?

"Roger's real dad gave him a new cap gun at the picnic yesterday. He wants to show it off," said Marlene.

The "real dad" of Roger was Marlene and Betty's real dad too; his name was Glen Gastor. You never saw him. You only heard about him. Harold Sadler would never let him on the place. The mother of the three kids was married to Harold Sadler and they also had a baby brother, Frank. Harold Sadler worked at USG but they also did some small scale farming like the Joneses and others. They would keep a cow and some chickens. A few hogs. Roger smelled bad from being around hogs. Dolores was a real Sadler. The other kids were Gastors but they were adopted and forced to call themselves "Sadler." It was very complicated. Hostility boiled up from Marlene.

David went up to Roger. "That's a great gun," he said. "Can I see it?"

"No," said Roger. "You'll break it."

"No I won't," David protested.

"See my ribbon," Marlene interrupted, pointing to the blue ribbon pinned to her blouse. "I won the gunny sack race yesterday. Don't forget it," she said.

"Somebody tripped me or I would have won," said Kate. They were talking about the United States Gypsum Labor Day Picnic at Olsen Park in Fort Dodge. The troupe moved on down the road with Kate leading. All nine of them were talking at once.

A quarter mile ahead they could see Sam and Lyle Evans's place at the corner. They would all turn north to the school from the Evanses' corner. Sam was going into Eighth with Kate. Sam wore a straw cowboy hat because he was a stable boy for Oren Gray in the afternoon. Lyle was five years old and starting Primary. Lyle talked all the time. Lyle's mother was not with them to see them off. She was probably drunk, David thought. That is what they all said. Everyone also said she hated Lyle and that Old Sam was not Sam's real dad. Someone would mention Sam's swarthy skin, and then you would hear someone mutter "nigger" and then someone would laugh, and it made David feel angry and it hurt Sam if he heard it. It all went back to when the Hills were full of coal mines and some of the miners were Negroes. He liked the word "swarthy," though.

The Evanses' yard was one massive junk pile with old cars, rusted bed springs, dilapidated, rotting furniture, and piles of cans and bottles, but no empty beer bottles. Beer bottles were worth a penny each. Old Sam Evans worked at USG and did some farming. He was very drunk at the USG picnic yesterday, people said. The previous day had been Labor Day, and all the kids whose dads worked at USG went to the USG picnic. David could not go to the picnic because his dad taught history and civics at Fort Dodge High School. He also coached football. David was proud of his dad.

Everyone waited for Sam and Lyle to come out. They could see the Harrises and Jordisons who were coming a ways off to the east. Jimmy, Larry and Mike Jordison are not related to Miss Jordison, but they liked her anyway. Sam came out and he was grinning like always. Lyle, his little brother, followed behind, talking. Sam was smart and strong and responsible. He had swarthy skin and he never had sunburn and he talked about getting on the Highway Patrol, but he always ignored his little brother, Lyle.

Sam was good friends with Bruce Pingle, who lived north of the school. Bruce was in Eighth.

Sam waved at Shorty Harris who was in Sixth and following Jimmy Jordison who was leading the group. Shorty was fat, a bully, and a coward and he was afraid of Jimmy Jordison who would beat him up if he bullied the little kids too much. Jimmy was in Eighth and the Jordisons were all Catholics with their own mystical powers. In their home they had pictures of Jesus with some kind of heart showing. They each wore a crucifix, and David always wished Methodists could wear a crucifix, but that was against the rules.

Shorty Harris and his older sister Donna went to a Community Church in Kalo, the village south of Coalville. Shorty said Catholics are not Christians, but he never said it in front of Jimmy. Shorty also said Pentecostals were not Christians. His sister Donna was in Seventh and she was smart, dark skinned, and she was a great singer. She sang "What Wondrous Love is This?" sometimes. She was starting to show breasts, but you were not supposed to notice. She was Mary in the Christmas Program last year. Bruce Pingle was Joseph. Joan Jones was the Angel on High last year, but she had finished Eighth and we did not know if Marlene would make a good

Angel on High because she was angry a lot. Joan Jones had been the perfect Angel on High.

The Jordisons and Harrises merged with Kate's group. "Roger Sadler has a cap gun," Shorty said loudly, pointing. "You aren't allowed to have cap guns in school. I think I'll take it away from him."

"No you won't," Marlene Sadler said, threateningly.

"No you won't," Jimmy Jordison said at the identical moment. "That's up to Miss Jordison. Shorty Harris, you shut up." He shut.

David and Roger ran over to meet Larry Jordison, who was going into Third, and his little brother Mike, who was going into First. Roger quick-drew his cap gun and fired on Larry Jordison. Larry grabbed his gut. Gut-shot, he bent over and collapsed onto his left shoulder. His leg jutted out straight and twitched. Then he wanted to look at Roger's cap gun, but we were all moving on toward school. Theatrics would have to wait.

Larry had his own death scene memorized, but Mike didn't even try, and kids wanted to tease him. Nobody ever bothered Mike even though he was slow in school, but he did not know how to die right when we pantomimed the cowboy movies. Jimmy saw to it that nobody teased Mike. Everyone protected Mike.

"You should have seen me at the picnic yesterday," Larry said to David and Roger. "I won the race. I beat a bunch of city slicker kids from Fort Dodge. Look!" He was wearing a blue ribbon with a golden paper badge inscribed with "First Place 50 Yard Dash United States Gypsum Picnic Labor Day 1950."

"Wow," said David. "Can I see it?"

"No," said Larry, "You'll ruin it."

"Come on," said Kate. She was the leader by default because her older sister Joan had finished the Eighth Grade last spring. They followed her up the road north from the Evans place a quarter mile to the school. Everyone sensed she was the new leader. David had loved Joan, but Kate was in charge of fifteen people now.

They reached Holliday Creek School and Jack Gorelle watched them arrive. He was the elected School Director. He was also the maintenance man, boss of the PTA, and a Democrat. He was repairing the pump that had been pulled out of the ground and lay on its side like a great big rusty tinker toy, David thought. The pump was in the southwest corner of the playground. Jack Gorelle was watching everyone, and everyone saw him, but no one waved to him like they did to Oren Gray. Jack Gorelle wore blue overalls and a blue shirt with a salt-stained pinstripe railroad engineer's cap with brown workman's brogans. A red bandanna hung out of his hip pocket. If you got close you would have seen he needed a shave; a slight trickle of tobacco juice oozed from the corner of his mouth.

To the north they saw more kids coming and they knew it was the tall lanky frame of Bruce Pingle leading his group. The Pingles owned farms. David could make out Wanda Mae Wilwhite and her brother Chester, who was going into Third. Darrel, Ronnie, and Christine Smith were coming too. Everyone had a lunch pail and a sack full of supplies. As they neared the school, they saw that Marsha Stein was already in the school yard talking to Miss Jordison. Marsha never walked to school. Her mom always drove her.

"There's Marsha Stein, already polishing the apple," Kate said. The ranks behind her agreed. The two groups did not arrive at the same time. Bruce Pingle's group of five came first and they stood by the gate and yelled hellos to Kate Jones and her fifteen. All twenty-four of us were back together, and we all mingled around. The first day of school was a reunion. We surrounded Miss Jordison. We were glad to see her.

This was the student roster of the Holliday Creek School:

Eighth Grade: Kate Jones, Sam Evans, Jimmy
    Jordison, Bruce Pingle
Seventh Grade: Marlene Sadler, Donna Harris
Sixth Grade: Shorty Harris, Betty Sadler
Fifth Grade: nobody
Fourth Grade: Janette Jones, Marsha Stein,
    Christine Smith, Francis Benson
Third Grade: David Wright, Roger Sadler, Larry
    Jordison, Chester Wilwhite, Ronnie Smith
Second Grade: Wanda Mae Wilwhite, Darrel Smith
First Grade: Walt Benson, Dolores Sadler, Mike
    Jordison
Primary: Lyle Evans

The First Day

We were twenty-three all together, and we surrounded Miss Jordison. She said, "This is the first day of school and we are all here." She smiled broadly, looked to the sky, raised her hands, palms up, and said, "We are all here, Lord." She shook the long dark curls on her shoulders and repeated the words. We all looked up.

She pointed to little Walt Benson, who had the cast on his arm. "I am glad to see you, Walt. How is your arm?"

Walt was embarrassed. He did not want to talk. "I fell," he said. "I fell." The kids looked at one another because they had heard otherwise. If Miss Jordison noticed it she would look into it, we thought.

Miss Jordison turned her attention to Bruce Pingle. "Bruce, we are going to say the Pledge and sing "Our Country, 'Tis of Thee." Would you go inside and get the flag? You know where it is." Bruce Pingle went inside the school. She had us form a circle around the flagpole. We did this every year the first day of school.

"Do you want us arranged according to grades?" Kate Jones asked.

Miss Jordison had not thought of that. "Yes," she said letting it become her idea. "Will you help arrange the students into grades?"

"Yes Miss Jordison," Kate replied. She took charge, but others helped.

Bruce Pingle came out with the flag. Miss Jordison nodded to him. He knew what to do, and he clipped the flag onto the rope and pulleyed it to the top of the flagpole. While he raised the flag, Miss Jordison said, "You boys take off your caps. Hold them over your hearts." We did. Nobody giggled or played horse. It was a very solemn moment. She had a good strong soprano voice and she started us off.

> My country, 'tis of thee,
> Sweet land of liberty, of thee I sing;

Others joined in.

> Land where my fathers died,
> Land of the pilgrims' pride,
> From every mountainside let freedom ring!

We always sang two verses. Some of us knew the words by heart. "The Star Spangled Banner" was too hard to sing.

> Our fathers' God, to thee,
> Author of liberty, to thee we sing;
> Long may our land be bright
> With freedom's holy light;
> Protect us by thy might, great God, our King.

The kids in Primary looked mystified, so while we sang Betty Sadler bent down near Lyle Evans and sang in his face while she held his hands. Kate Jones put her arm around Mike Jordison, who was in First, but he couldn't remember the words from last year.

Miss Jordison said, "Jimmy Jordison, would you lead us in the Pledge?" Jimmy's dad had a small farm and did not work in the mills. Jimmy stepped out in the center forgetting all this. He was embarrassed to speak, but he said,

> I pledge a legion to the flag
> Of the United States of American
> And to the public for which it stands
> One nation, invisible
> With liberty and judges for all.

The kids all recited what he said right after he said it. It was like an echo. Most did not know the words. They just echoed what they thought he said.

Miss Jordison did not scold him, but nodded and smiled at Jimmy. David wanted to correct him, but kept still. David's Dad had taught him all the words to the Pledge and their meanings when he was still in First. David recited them correctly, he thought, but Jimmy was the leader right then so he shut up.

"All right," said Miss Jordison, looking toward the top of the flagpole. "This is the American flag." The wind was out of the west, It was going to get hot soon. "And the flag stands for us all. It has forty eight stars. One for each state. Our state is Iowa. Who knows the motto for our state?" She looked over at Marlene Sadler and nodded.

Marlene said, "Our liberties we prize and our rights we will maintain." She remembered that from last year. We all remembered how hard she worked to memorize that line for our Armistice Day Ceremony the year before. That was because her real dad was a war veteran and he fought the Germans, and he was at the school to accept some kind of award from J. Clare Robinson himself, the County Superintendent of Schools. That was the only time anyone had seen Mr. Gastor. He was a hero. Marlene had memorized the words. We all remembered when she didn't remember when practicing her line last year, but she got it right during the ceremony. Today she remembered. Miss Jordison continued.

"America is a democracy and that means the people are important. We can vote in this country. Men and women can vote. Some people say women should not vote, but men who say that are ignorant. Only men say that. Women do not say that. We will be having an election for School Director in November and everyone needs to vote. Tell your mothers they need to come to the school board meeting and vote."

While she spoke, Jack Gorelle had moved in close to listen. He wore blue overalls and a blue shirt with a pinstripe railroad engineer's cap with brown workman's brogans. A red bandanna hung out of his hip pocket. He needed a shave. A slight trickle of tobacco juice emerged from the corner of his mouth. He was the "Director" elected by the parents in the community. He was not County Superintendent. That was J. Claire Robinson. Jack Gorelle was watching the goings-on the first day of school.

"What is our state motto, everyone?" said Miss Jordison. She raised her left hand, palm upward, signifying we were to recite aloud.

"Our liberties we prize and our rights we will maintain," some of us said, a little off guard.

"That's right. One of our liberties is the right to vote. For women as well as for men. One of our rights is the right to belong to a union. I guess you heard about that at the USG Picnic yesterday." Many students' fathers worked for United States Gypsum company and they were in the union. She continued. "Another liberty is public education. We will maintain the right to an education this year. We all need to be educated, so we all have to help educate one another. I can't teach everything to everybody, so we have to go by the idea of Each One Teach One. That is part of democracy." The tone of her voice changed. *"Education is the idea that everybody knows something important that somebody else doesn't know, so you share what you know rather than leave them in the dark.* You all know how it works. At Holliday Creek School we help one another.

"I see most of you have brought your supplies. We are going inside now, so you need to sit according to grade. Each person has a desk to keep supplies in. There is a file card with your name on it at each desk. Jimmy, Bruce, Kate, Sam, Marlene, Betty, can you help? You know what to do. Are there any questions?"

Shorty Harris said, "Roger Sadler has a cap gun . . ." But she cut him off.

"Don't be a tattletale, Shorty," she said. "I saw he has a cap gun in a fine new holster. Roger, I want to talk to you after everyone goes in. Go inside now, everyone."

Everyone headed inside, except Miss Jordison and Roger Sadler, who had his chin on his chest. Miss Jordison looked at Jack Gorelle, who was watching. "Mr. Gorelle, are you repairing the pump or acting as director, prying into the workings of the school?" she asked, putting her hand under Roger's chin and lifting it.

"Yes I am, Miss Jordison," he said, agreeing to both. "That speech was very good. Yer mention of the election for Director and all. Too bad yer dad can't run for Director, but he lives out of District." She knew he was smirking as he returned to the pump. She thought about this. *He did not care a hoot about Roger Sadler, but he knew Roger's dad was in jail along with his medals. Mr. Sadler could not hurt him. Jack Gorelle had been told to fix the pump during the summer, but here it was the first day of school and the pump still did not work, but what did that that matter? He was elected Director, and the pump would be working by election time.*

The school had no water. Bruce Pingle and Jimmy Jordison watched her talking to Jack Gorelle. They knew they did not have more than one bucket of water, but they did not want to scare the little kids. Bruce and Jimmy would talk about it tonight at the supper table, you could be sure.

Meanwhile the kids filed inside the school, and as they did they heard Kate say in a falsetto: "Tattletale, tattletale hanging on a bull's tail; When the bull begins to pee Shorty gets a cup of tea."

Everyone sort of laughed except for Shorty, who glared at anyone who giggled. David laughed. Shorty heard him. "I'll get even for that," Shorty said. Kids were always saying they were going to get even. David felt panicky for a second, but he figured he was okay as long as Kate was around. She had slapped Shorty silly last year. Kate knew the "justice for all" part. David started unloading his sack of supplies like everyone else.

*   *   *

It was lunch time. And Miss Jordison dismissed the class. They could eat anywhere but were forbidden to leave the yard. That was why they noticed Sam Evans and Bruce Pingle walking up the road to the Faust farm with water pails.

Long ago, Bob Jordison's father had deeded an acre of land to the county to use for a school. They had named it "Holliday Creek School." Miss Jordison was really Eleanor Faust, but the students refused to call her Mrs. Faust even after she and Jake got married last year. She remained Miss Jordison to the students forever and ever. Jake did not seem to mind. He always smiled in every situation. Sam Evans and Bruce Pingle were after water because Jack Gorelle had not fixed the school pump. As School Director, Jack Gorelle had hired himself to do well maintenance that he did not do. Bruce said to Sam he figured Jack Gorelle ought to be arrested. Sam agreed.

Younger boys gathered in the northwest corner of the school yard near the big oak tree. It was hot. Jack Gorelle had torn down their fort and burned it near the tree. The ash pile was evidence, and they hated him for that. "Fire hazard," he had said. He was not working on the pump because he had gone home. The boys sat down and began to talk about how they would rebuild the fort. While they talked they opened their lunch pails. Darrel Smith called it a lunch bucket. They argued over that. They argued a lot. Usually Larry and David were on the same side. They said it was a pail. Chester Wilwhite and Ronny Smith were on the other side saying it was a lunch bucket. Roger Sadler was always deciding which side to take. He was a swing vote. Today he decided it was a lunch pail. While they argued they bartered lunch *pail* items. No decision was made about the fort.

Soon Sam and Bruce returned with the water pails. They filled the crockery jug in the basement. It had a spigot. Each kid had a paper Dixie Cup to drink out of. Students each got a new Dixie Cup every week. They quit using the old water pail and dipper when Miss Jordison took over as teacher. She said a dipper was unsanitary. Jack Gorelle was against Dixie Cups. "Too sissified," was his comment. "'Sides, they cost money. Too much spending." He never said "besides."

The first day of school was ending and everything was put away. Each student had a task. The blackboard was erased and the floor was swept. The trash was taken out and burned. Sam and Bruce went out with the water pails and headed for the Faust farm so we would have water in the morning. Usually they went to the pump in the school yard, but Jack Gorelle was gone and the pump was lying on the concrete slab still unfixed.

David's job was to empty the pencil sharpener, and he decided that graphite is very smooth between the fingers. The graphite felt like oil. He played with the pine wood and graphite shavings. His fingers were black, but he did not notice it.

Each row had to be inspected as students stood by their desks. Miss Jordison would say, "You may pass." And when she said it they walked to the door. It was all very orderly until they got outside. Then they broke into groups yelling like Indians or whooping like cowboys. The Jones-Jordison-Evans group headed south and the Pingle group headed north. They waved good-bye. It was hot, and David could feel the heavy starch in his denim overalls melting to stick on his thighs. He was sweating and his sweat still felt like Rose Hair Dressing running down his face. He wiped his hand over his sweating face. He was spreading graphite all over his face and did not realize it.

Larry was sprinting down the road and David ran to catch up with him. When Larry stopped, he looked back and saw David's face. It was mostly black. Larry laughed. He fell down laughing. Everyone caught up to them and they saw David with his blackened face. "Nigger, nigger, nigger," Shorty Harris howled. He had gotten even. Sam Evans did not laugh as he walked by. He would get even.

Janette said, "David, you look a fright." She showed him his reflection in her compact mirror she kept in the pocket of her dress. He was impossible. She waltzed off.

It did not matter how hard he sweated by the time he got home. Sweat would never wash off the graphite. They would never forget the black graphite on his face. Everyone in the school would laugh about it. For years. Actually, he thought it was funny, too, and he would have made a bigger Al Jolson scene of it but he was tired and he had chores to do. Most of them had chores to do when they got home except for Marcia Stein, he supposed. He lagged behind the Jones girls on ahead as everyone turned off to their homes. David was thinking things over.

He was no different from others, but Roger smelled bad from being around pigs, while a person never smelled bad from being around lambs, David thought. He had the lambs to care for along with Johnny. He had to get home. The lambs would be hungry. He always fed his lambs. It had been a good day. David felt a little sadness to leave Holliday Creek School and the boys he had not seen all summer, but he kept faith that they would be there tomorrow. The Jones girls were far ahead when David encountered and stopped to look at a sheaf of Boxelder branches lying broken and wilted alongside the road.

The One Room School House

If you had attended Holliday Creek School, you would have noticed all the desks faced south. On the first day of school each kid found his or her desk marked with a file card. They all started unloading their bags of stuff into the desks. Desks were curlicue black cast iron with a wooden desk top. There was a wooden shelf under the slanted desk top and that is where they put school supplies. Most desk tops had letters gouged in them. You were forbidden to carve initials on a desk top, but initials got carved anyway. At the upper right corner of the desk top was an empty hole. The holes were for ink wells, but they did not use ink wells much anymore. They still used them during penmanship class.

David saw Janette was saying something snotty over her shoulder to Marsha Stein. Marsha had her nose in the air, showing disdain for Janette. Marsha had a huge box of crayons with four shades of each color. Ronny Smith saw her coloring box and said there should be a rule about anyone having more than one color of orange. "It's not fair," he said. Ronny Smith said "not fair" a lot.

Books were being passed out and students were trying to cram them into their desks. Most books were used and dog-eared, but David got a new speller and a penmanship notebook. There were posters on the wall showing the correct way to write cursive. David curled his lip because he hated penmanship. He practiced curling his lip. Bad guys in the movies were good at curling lips.

Miss Jordison's desk was in the southeast corner—the front of the room. Everyone was very direction-conscious. David sat more or less in the northwest corner—just off the northwest section of the classroom was the cloak room. Other people called it the coat room. They argued over that. Between the coat room and the stairwell was a narrow room with bookshelves. It was the storage room and library.

The south wall had lots of blackboard space and one window in the southwest corner that looked south along the road toward the Evans farm. The road ran south of that to Jack Gorelle's place. Everyone saw Jack Gorelle drive away. He was going home. No work would be done on the pump today. Everybody knew. It was like a nonverbal mass conclusion that rippled through the room. Miss Jordison saw him drive away, but said nothing. Then she looked out the windows along the east wall. The older kids sat along the east wall. They had a grand view of the cornfield and the grove of trees off to the east. But it was the coldest part of the school. Both registers were along the west wall where the little kids sat.

The furnace was in the basement in the boiler room. Adjacent to the boiler room on the south side was a room where corn cobs were kept. It was "the cob bin." Corn cobs were donated by farmers. It was Jack Gorelle's job to see that the school had plenty of corn cobs. He would shovel them through a chute. Corn cobs were used for starting the fire Monday mornings if the teacher did not do a good job banking the fire to keep the furnace lit over the week end. You could not heat the school with corn cobs. Next to the stair well was a coal bin. Jack Gorelle would shovel cannel coal down a chute and fill it in the fall. Coal still came out of the Hills. Older boys took turns checking on the furnace and shoveling coal during the school day. There always were arguments as to whether the school was too hot or too cold. Everyone had a sweater, and you could put it on or take it off to compensate. The smoke stank and ashes were a problem. There was no pot bellied stove and the students did not chop wood. The school had electricity, but there was no electrical pump. People had to pump water by hand and carry it in to the schoolhouse. Everyone was edgy because the pump was broken. They had to carry water from the Faust farm next door.

Gary Pingle and Lyle Evans turned to look out the east window when Miss Jordison looked out at her husband, Jake. Jake was out there fixing fence, but he had turned to look south—watching Jack Gorelle drive away, heading for home.

The Rules

Miss Jordison went over The Rules. As she did, she carried a yardstick and rapped on one desk or another as she paced up and down the aisles. It was for emphasis. She was never known to whack you with it, but you paid attention, anyway. She had a stick and she was not afraid to whip us. That included older boys, but if an older boy challenged her, she would simply expel you, they said—but no one ever got expelled. Once or twice a year someone got a couple whacks across the buttocks. She made sure it hurt. There was no flogging. Mostly we obeyed because she was Miss Jordison and this was school.

She wrote the rules on the blackboard.

- Girls could go to the toilet unaccompanied. Our toilets were outhouses.
- Boys in the Fourth grade and younger had to be accompanied by an older boy to see that they did not pee out behind the outhouse or on the seats.
- If you need to leave the room you were to raise your hand and ask if you could leave the room. (That was very embarrassing)
- You cannot bring cap guns or bb guns to school.
- Each person is to teach something to somebody every day.

- You could color in the coloring book during Reading Aloud, but you were not allowed to whisper or talk.
- If you do especially well you get to choose what game we will play at recess.
- Gum. Candy. Wastepaper. Talking out of turn.
- Dixie cups
- Clean-up chores

1. Who pumps water
2. Who carries out ashes
3. Who sweeps off mud
4. David will empty the pencil sharpener

- Snores

We started class after that.

Recess

In mid morning we would have recess. Today Donna Harris got to choose what all of us did on the playground that day because she was being rewarded for unpacking books. "Bat and Ball," she said. We never called the game "Baseball." City slicker kids called it baseball. Spike Jones called his musicians, the City Slickers, but we used the term more broadly and in a negative way. The older boys got the bat and ball from the equipment box. We had straw-filled canvas bags for the bases. Only a few of the boys had baseball gloves, and those who had them were apt to be called "sissy." Ronny Smith complained it was not fair that some kids had baseball gloves and others did not.

Girls played "Workup" along with the boys. On that day Betty Sadler was First Bat. Gary Pingle was Second Bat, and then came Third Bat and Fourth Bat. You could stay on as a batter until you flew out, struck out, got thrown out, or hit the ball over the fence. "Over the Fence is Out" was the wise ruling. If you were out, you had to go to right field. Everyone rotated with every out unless you flew out. If you flew out you traded positions with the person who caught your fly. The number of fielders was variable. If lots of kids stayed home sick, we would cut back on the number of fielders. It was a negotiated decision. Miss Jordison let us work it out. After a ground out, the pitcher became Fourth Bat and had to double as catcher.

The game never ended because there were no innings. No one kept score because there were no teams. Everyone memorized everyone's position when recess ended. The main objective was to get to bat and stay at bat. Eventually you had to get to bat. It was unavoidable. We all resumed the same positions the next time someone chose to play Bat and Ball. Miss Jordison called balls and strikes and decided if you were out or safe. In the previous year she had appointed Joan Jones to umpire while she watched the little ones playing. With Joan now in high school, everyone wondered who would be Umpire this year? The Umpire settled arguments and had the power to send you to the basement until recess was over. The Umpire had power.

On days we did not play Bat and Ball we played Pom Pom Pull Away. Or Fox and Geese. Or Kickball or Soccer. We would plan ahead knowing what game we would choose. You only got to choose if you did something outstanding. Smart kids got to choose most often.

Meanwhile, the little kids played in the sand box or in the swing or on the teeter totter or played cowboy or tag. At noon they played marbles or mumblety-peg or jump rope or hop scotch or jacks. After Third they were expected to play organized games.

Miss Jordison rang the hand bell. We always rushed for the door because someone was going to read aloud.

Reading Aloud

As a general policy, right after recess Miss Jordison would have one of the students read fiction to us. It developed listening skills—part of which was to sit quiet. During Reading Aloud you could color in your coloring book. Or you could daydream. Or even sleep. But you could not talk or even whisper. Hand signals were forbidden. If you disturbed the reading, you had to sit in the basement. The separation from the class was a formidable threat, so you listened. Most of us enjoyed Reading Aloud, so there was considerable peer pressure. Listening was a good skill that carried over from school to church or Scout meetings or PTA meetings.

I learned to love fiction. The boys tended to like the Hardy Boys mysteries and western stories. Jack London was the favorite author. We read *Call of the Wild* and *White Fang*. My other favorites were Laura Ingalls Wilder books. Everyone was touched when Mary went blind.

Miss Jordison let us choose the next book. "Book Reports" were advocacy sessions for books we had read ourselves and that we loved so much we were willing to read them aloud. Sometimes we convinced other people to read a story and they would do a book report on the same story. Like the story *To Build a Fire*. Students also decided who would be Reader, so just because you made a good book report you did not automatically get to read it aloud. I practiced reading *To Build a Fire,* but I never got to read it aloud to the school.

The Reader was expected to read the story like a radio program, especially when it came to dialogue. You changed voices when you were reading the narrative. You changed tones and did accents when you were reading dialogue. You improvised. I began inserting sound effects, mentally, like listening to a radio program. I could mimic Sergeant Preston of the Yukon pretty well. I never became a speed reader for that reason.

During Reading Aloud Miss Jordison could grade papers or plan things. She could do that and listen at the same time.

Student Empowerment

For lessons in different subjects, most of the time Miss Jordison would gather a small group around her desk and kids would recite. We were generally grouped according to reading level or math level, not necessarily by grade. You could listen in on the lesson. When the Upper Graders recited their history lessons, I listened in and mouthed the words Vasco da Gama well enough that Jimmy Jordison could glance over and read my lips and get the right answer. Jimmy was answering the question about "Who tried to open a trade route to India?" I remembered hearing the recitation during past years. I knew Jimmy was grateful, and Jimmy would keep Shorty from getting even with me when I laughed at him. That was how the system worked.

Miss Jordison was a master at classroom management, and she first introduced us to the idea of student empowerment, following the idea of Each One Teach One. She delegated and that way she *diffused* her power. While she worked with a small group of students around her desk, other groups were at work. For instance, a Sixth-grade girl like Betty Sadler would oversee Second and Third graders as they did their math assignment. Betty was a born math teacher. Everybody, particularly Miss Jordison, was quick to see it. Meanwhile, Betty was doing her own math problems at the same time. The highest level of understanding a subject is being able to teach it. Betty had the right to decide if you had done your math. If you didn't do your work, Betty had the power keep you in from recess. Nobody made fun of her buck teeth. Each One Teach One, therefore, broke the teacher's monopoly of power.

Jimmy Jordison was in charge of the Middle Grade history, but he couldn't teach. His brother Larry and I would help him find places on a map. We would get kids to read aloud, and we would explain things to Ronnie Smith and Chester Wilwhite. We all worked out the right answers to the questions. Roger Sadler daydreamed a lot.

At home, Dad monitored my progress, and asked me lots of questions about school. He could have hauled me to town and enrolled me at Carpenter School where he was principal but he decided against it. Instead, he monitored my progress against the city kids. He brought home spelling books and reading books from Carpenter School. I took tests. He could see I was reading two or three years ahead of the same class in Fort Dodge. Math was about the same. Verbal skills were off the chart. He thought it was remarkable that a system with one teacher for eight grades could work.

Miss Jordison used lessons that had been prepared by many teachers at our school over the years. Students recognized them from last year and the year before. Lesson plans got refined and passed down from succeeding teachers. It was educational evolution in action.

Old Jim

Dad first met Jim Jones right after we bought the farm. Dad was remodeling the kitchen. Old Jim walked into the yard and they talked.

"What do you do?" Old Jim asked.

"I teach history and civics at the high school," Dad said.

"A professor." Jim Jones knew Dad was not a professor, but he had a way of turning your advantage back upon you so that you would have to defend it.

That is how Old Jim got my dad to say, "No, I am not a professor, but I have my degree from the University of Minnesota. What do you do, Mr. Jones?"

"I'm a flunky at USG but I am in good with the union steward." Jim Jones spit between the toes of his shoes. He was a Democrat, of course. He and his wife, Maudie, had three daughters living at home. The boys were Jimmy and Dick. Jimmy was off on his own. We referred to them as young Jim and Old Jim.

Joan was the oldest of the girls. She was starting Eighth grade, her last year at Holliday Creek School. When this topic came up with Old Jim, Dad said,

"Then she will be going to high school next year."

Old Jim was against it. "Girls have no goddamn business going to school beyond the Eighth grade," he declared, spitting tobacco juice between his feet. He dipped snuff, but he did not smoke because that was unhealthy. Smoke was just as bad for the lungs as coal dust or gypsum dust. People in the Hills knew about Black Lung. It was a message that had been passed on down. He said, "None of us ever went beyond the Eighth grade. No need to. What's a woman need with more education?" That ended the discussion.

Dad repeated his words often. Dad could not grasp how anyone could have such low self-esteem and hold such a low opinion of education. Dad would say, "Old Jim could have said, 'I work at United States Gypsum,' or 'I'm a maintenance man,' or something, but to refer to yourself as a 'flunky' is beyond belief. Sometimes people need to depreciate themselves for no good reason." Dad was very wise.

Mom would say, "Maybe he's modest."

Old Jim could be an obliging neighbor. During the first year on Holliday Creek, he was willing to lend a hand and a mechanic's skill, such as when he and Dad installed the new furnace at our place.

Dad knew how to hang duct work and install a furnace because Granddad Wright was a tin smith in Audubon, Iowa, the town where my dad grew up. Dad always helped his father hang downspouts or install furnaces and ducts.

Old Jim was impressed that Dad knew how to install a furnace, connect the duct work, and install the registers. Old Jim was generous to a fault. He refused any payment for the water we took from his spring that was up on the side of the hill, on the other side of a fence. To get to the spring you had to climb a stile, which was a set of wooden steps that crossed over the fence. The stile that was there was rotting and rickety. It needed replacing. Old Jim allowed Dad to pay for the building materials when they worked together and built a new stile. "A man must allow others to draw water from the well," Old Jim said. He would say that often.

"Dick Wright, I have to admit you are not a total city slicker," Old Jim would say, grinning. "You are a pretty good carpenter." Then he would spit between his shoes. Dad was all right in his book.

Dad, as well, knew he had a good neighbor and that they could work together, but Dad knew what he was up against when I finished my first year in Holliday Creek and it came time to help Joan Jones get a high school diploma. Dad discussed it with Mom, who said, "Leave it to me." She intended to talk to Mrs. Jones.

Now, Maudie Jones was a beautiful woman in her forties, and she was worldly wise. Old Jim was ten or twelve years her senior. Her sons, Jimmy and Dick, were older than Joan, Catherine, and Janette. Her sons had jobs with USG. Their education ended at Holliday Creek School. Maudie wanted her girls to have a high school education. We knew this because she liked my mom and she would walk up the lane to our house bringing fresh baked rolls. They would visit. Maudie was not heavy, but she was not slim. Men would notice her, like when there was a PTA meeting at the school or she was in the grocery in Coalville. She told Mom, "I can get Jim to let Joan go to school. I know how to get men to do what I want. I learned to do that when I was young."

Mom knew what she meant, and Old Jim was not a tyrant, so the day after Labor Day, 1948, we waved to Joan as she walked by our place to catch the school bus at Bob Jordison's place on top of the Hill. I need to proclaim how radiant she was with her strawberry blond hair and tanned skin. How confident she was. How shy. How determined and eventually how triumphant! It would be her *first day* of high school and some barriers were about to fall.

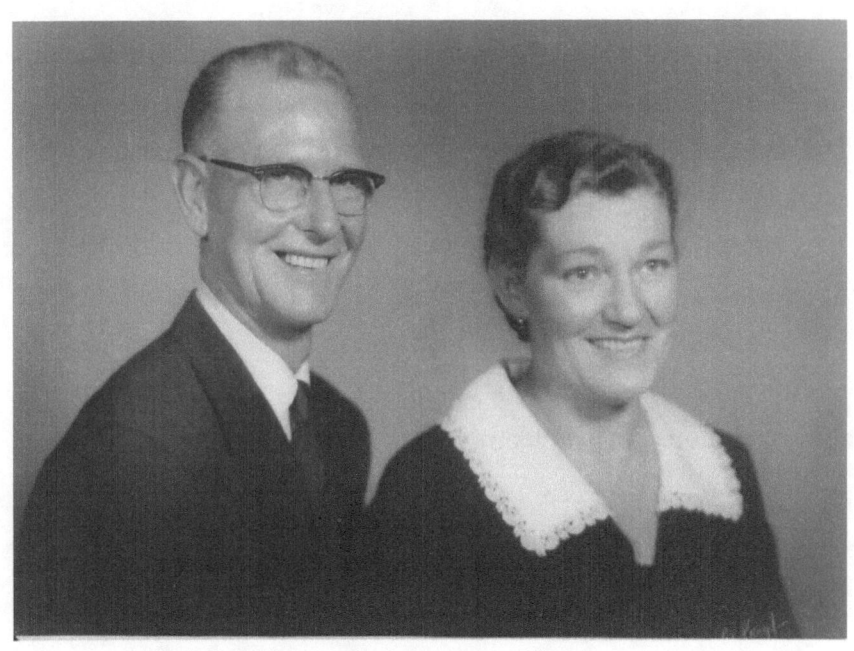

Jim and Maudie Jones

Saturday

It was 2:45 p.m. on a Saturday and my family was headed home from Fort Dodge. The day had been well planned. It had started in Fort Dodge that morning when Dad had dropped Mom and us boys off at the public library at nine o'clock.

Our Saturdays usually followed a familiar pattern. After Dad dropped us off, he went to the bank. At the library we checked out lots of books. We did not have many books at school, but the public library was a bonanza. Mom and Dad read too, but not as much as they did before we had electricity and a radio.

Mom would go to the Women's Club meeting. One time she told me about a wonderful little girl pianist named Polly Kaderabek. She talked about how she played beautiful music from Debussy. Mom played our piano and she had Dad bring home some records from school. We had a Victrola. Mom decided I should learn to play the piano too, so she bought some books for beginning piano students from the music store and tried to teach me to play. She tried to get the Jones girls to play too.

Some Saturdays she went to the Blandon Memorial Art Gallery. Mom herself was one who drew, wrote and painted. She also belonged to the Art Guild and a writer's club. Meanwhile, Dad would take Johnny and me to the high school with him to swim. He kept keys even though he no longer taught there. He was promoted to principal at Carpenter School. Dad took us swimming even in winter. The kids at Holliday Creek School thought that swimming was good, but they always thought Dad was a city slicker and that I was bragging.

Other Saturdays, Dad took us to Kautzky's sporting good store to buy fishing hooks, sinkers, or BBs. Kautzky's always had sporting goods only the rich could buy, but it was fun to look and wish. After we swam or shopped we would stop at the Maid-Right for, believe it or not, Maid-Rights. Then Johnny and I went to the matinee. We got to choose the movie. Usually we saw a western. Movies during the late 1940s were an experience in and of themselves.

While we watched the movie, Mom and Dad shopped.

Johnny and I waited in front of the theater after the movie. We were allowed to walk up and down the block until my parents arrived—under the watchful eye of the green clock tower of downtown Fort Dodge. We could look in the different shops, but we were not allowed to cross the street because Richard got run over by a car crossing the street. We were by ourselves until they picked us up.

Saturdays were wonderful. Then on Sundays we had to get up and drive back into town for church. Sundays were never as much fun. All the stores were closed. Movies were forbidden for us on Sunday because we were Methodists. Catholics could go to the movies on Sundays, but Catholics were Democrats and they drank too.

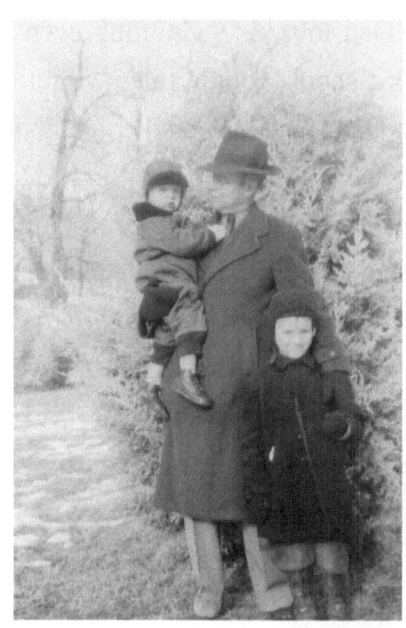
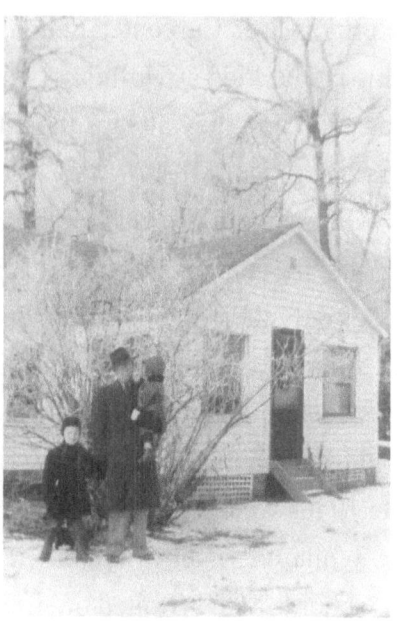
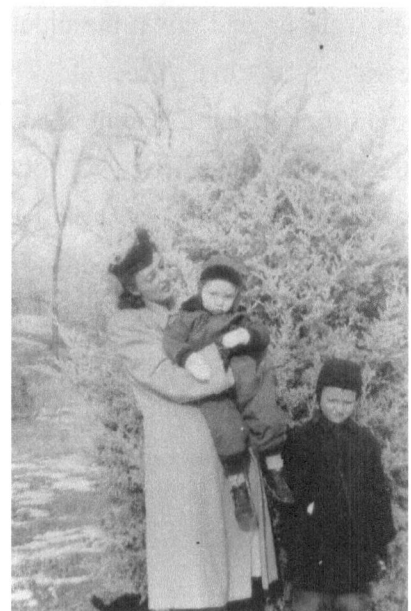

Frosty Sunday Morning

On our way home on Saturdays, we would sometimes meet the Joneses driving toward town in their new Pontiac. We waved back and forth. Our day was ending, but theirs was just starting.

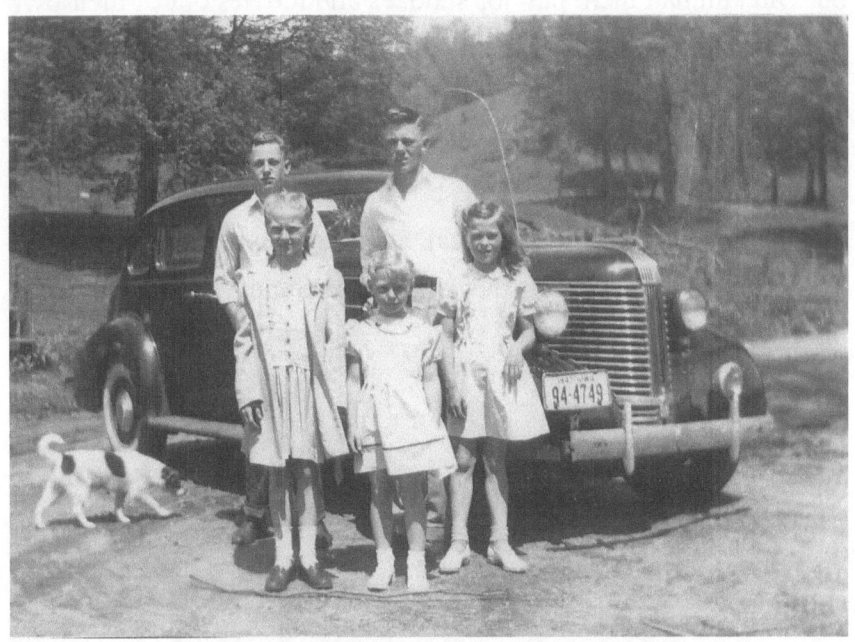

Jones's 1947 Pontiac
Back: Dick, Jimmy
Front: Joan, Janette, Kate

On Saturdays, Maudie got her girls ready to go shopping. Old Jim would work until noon to get overtime. Then he would go home, take a bath, and drive his family to town. Old Jim liked Pontiacs. Maudie could find bargains on clothes so her girls looked good and never did without. Then they went shopping for groceries, and then to the Maid-Right. The Maid-Right had parking places at night when they were closed. The Joneses would park their car there and take the girls to the movies. First they would get sundaes at The Dutch Mill. The girls got to choose the movie. Sometimes they would split up and go to different theaters. The Jones girls had a lot of freedom, but Old Jim had them pay for sundaes and movies out of their own pockets. No handouts for them. Then Maudie and Jim would go to the I.O.O.F. Dance up above Fantle's Department Store, featuring live music. When the movie was over, the girls would meet their parents at the dance. The Joneses enjoyed the dance. In their car, they had blankets in the back seat, and they slept on the way home. They could sleep as late as they wanted on Sundays. That was a day of rest.

The American Dream

It was February and Jerry Smith and I were playing in The Hills on a Sunday afternoon. We decided to sneak up on his older brother Norman and Dick Jones. They were holed up at the old tool shed that was called the shack. The shack was up toward the top of the hill where there was an old abandoned mineshaft. Janette and I had gone back into the mineshaft many times even though we were forbidden to play there. Bats lived in the mineshaft. You could look down on Holliday Creek from the shack and see Oren Gray's barn. Jerry and I climbed the steep ravine toward the shack.

Dick Jones and Norman Smith had rejuvenated the tool shed, sort of. They were teenagers without much money, so they collected cast-off chairs and a table and they patched the roof. They even found panes of glass for the window and built bunks. There was a sheet-metal stove and a blue coffee pot. It was not much of a place but it was their place, or so they thought. Norman and Dick slept there some weekends and hatched plans for a bank robbery. They would buy cars with the loot. Dick liked Pontiacs but he would settle for a Dodge. Norman wanted a Cadillac. He aspired for more. They had bread, peanut butter, and jelly. They also had cigarette papers and "Bull" Durham tobacco. They knew how to do a roll-your-own cigarette.

Nothing much took place up there, except I tried tobacco. I could not get the hang of rolling a cigarette, though.

Coalmining in Webster County (Part One)

By Roger Natte

[Author's Note: This essay on coal and coal miners is excerpted with permission from a 2001 article of the same name appearing at a website on Coalville, Iowa, the place described in this book. Roger Natte is an expert on the history of Fort Dodge, a city near Coalville in Webster County, Iowa. This material draws upon his research.]

The Development of Iowa Coal

The genesis of Iowa coal is found in the geological era known as the Pennsylvanian period, which began over two hundred fifty million years ago and lasted some fifty million years. This was a period in which the unique conditions required for the formation of coal were met on a grand scale. Coal is an accumulation of plant material in the form of peat, which has been subjected to pressure and heat. The first condition necessary for its creation is the prolific growth of vegetation. Experts estimate that under model conditions it takes twenty feet of plant material to compress into three feet of peat, which in turn can produce one foot of coal. The time needed to produce that much plant material is three thousand years. Since mineable coal in Webster County ranges from two and one half to ten feet in thickness, between fifty and two hundred feet of plant material would be required, needing between 7,500 and 30,000 years to accumulate. An additional 25,000 to 100,000 years is necessary to transform that material into coal.

The Coalville district, one of the county's largest, measures about two and three-quarters miles long and one and three-quarters mile wide. In that field a unique seam, the "big coal," sometimes reaching a thickness of ten feet, is in long strips, two hundred to three hundred feet wide, which curves through the area, possibly a result of the marsh developing in the bed of an old river. In most cases the coal deposit takes a lens shape, with the thickest coal in the center of the field and feathering out toward the edges.

Coal has several forms; anthracite, bituminous, cannel, and lignite. Anthracite or hard coal, and lignite or brown coal, are not found in Webster County. The local coal is primarily of the bituminous variety, which is soft and breaks easily. It contains a large percentage of volatile materials, burns with a strong yellowish flame, leaving considerable ash, and gives off dense smoke. (Local pioneer lore tells that the early settlers first used local coal to produce smoke to keep mosquitoes away.) A few mines, primarily around Kalo, produced cannel coal. Its high number of BTUs makes it desirable for both the gypsum mills and the clay products plants in the area. Cannel coal also contains more ash material than other coal. Often when the volatile materials burned and the gases were driven off, the cannel coal ash expanded greatly, giving rise to the settlers' claim that if you burned a bushel of cannel coal you had to carry out a bushel and one half of ash, a claim that may not have been far from the truth. Webster County historically has had five coal producing areas: the Coalville-Kalo-Holliday Creek district, the Lehigh district, the Skillet Creek district east of Dayton, all of which are on or near the Des Moines River, and the Tara district on Lizard Creek several miles west of Fort Dodge. Exposure of seams in the walls of the valleys and ravines of the streams allowed easy discovery and easy mining through slope and drift entries.

The Holliday Creek-Coalville District

The Holliday Creek-Coalville district in Pleasant Valley Township was to become the first extensive commercial mining development in the county and began with the extension of railroads into the county in 1869. The Holliday Creek coal deposits were ideal for development because they were within a few miles of the Illinois Central railroad line. The first of these railroad inspired companies was the Holliday Creek Railroad and Coal Company incorporated in March of 1870 by John F. Duncombe, C. B. Richards and Platt Smith, among others. A company town with company owned housing and a company store was established, at that time considered a very progressive action. Assessor's records of 1880 indicate that the company owned sixty-six houses along Holliday Creek for rental to its employees and a general store located in Coalville. Finally, an 1885 newspaper item indicates that the company operated a school with 122 pupils. The Company ruled with an iron hand and brooked no opposition from its employees as seen in its work rules, published in 1870. Anyone who was "of cross and complaining, or quarrelsome disposition or who incites strikes, or interferes with the manage(ment) of the company, as soon as found out will be discharged." And "any person discharged for cause will never under any circumstances be permitted to again work for the Company." And "every employee . . . expressly agrees that in case of injury or death, no action or right of action shall ever be maintained against the Company on account of such injury or death." The Fort Dodge Coal Company may well have been the county's biggest producer of coal over the history of the local industry. All of the mines were in the Coalville-Holliday Creek district with the exception of the Parle mine at Kalo in which the company had a financial interest. The number four mine was the most productive and longest operating mine in the county . . . In 1887 that mine alone employed 127 men. An idea as to the size of the total operation of the company can be seen in the 1886 Mining Inspector's Report which indicated that the company was using twenty horses and mules in its underground operations and two steam locomotives to haul coal from its mines to the railroad.

In 1887 Mine Number Four still appeared to be productive but the company had begun to sell its assets. Dissolution may have been decided upon because it was believed that the Holliday Creek-Coalville deposits were rapidly being depleted. Indeed, the last mine that the company opened, "Number Sixteen," had proven to be unproductive, largely because pockets of rock interrupted the coal seam, making mining difficult and expensive.

The Trunk

School was out and the Jones girls were thinking up things to do. An old trunk was in the corner of the garage and we opened it. There were some toys in there and a jar of marbles. There were some boy's clothes too. I realized it was Richard's stuff, but everyone was curious. There were his shoes. There were baby shoes and coloring books with pictures of pilots and bombers. Also a Tonette whistle pipe and a toothbrush.

Janette found a pale blue dress in there, sized for an adult. She pulled it out and held it up. "Beautiful dress," Joan said, and she took it from Janette. Kate watched. Joan held the dress out at arm's length, admiring. Then she slipped it over her head.

Just about then Mom walked in, with Johnny. Mom sort of gasped at the scene. She gathered herself, and gesturing toward the children's items said, "These are Richard's things."

Joan said, "Who is Richard?"

"He was my brother," I said. We understood the moment.

Mom said, "I think we will put them away for now." She was not angry. "Richard was killed." She pulled an old newspaper out of the trunk, an issue of *The Advocate-Republican* from Thursday, February 1, 1945, and read from the front page.

Young Boy Fatally
Injured Thursday

Six-Year-Old Son of Mr. and

Mrs. J. R. Wright Jr. of

Fort Dodge Is Killed

Graveside services for Richard Dale Wright, six year-old son of Mr. and Mrs. J. R. Wright Jr. of Fort Dodge will be held at Arlington Heights cemetery in Audubon at two o'clock Saturday afternoon.

Richard was fatally injured Thursday noon when he was struck by a car as he was crossing the intersection in front of his home. Richard was returning home from school for lunch when the accident occurred.

He was born in Anamosa, Iowa on April 16, 1938.

He is survived by his parents and one brother, David, two years old. His grandparents, Mr. and Mrs. J. R. Wright, and Aunt Mary Wright reside in Audubon. A twin sister, Rose Mary, preceded him in death in infancy.

Funeral services will be held in Fort Dodge Saturday morning at ten o'clock. The Rev. C. H. Orf of the Audubon Methodist church will be in charge of the graveside services here.

She said, "He was a twin. His sister was Rose Mary. She died the day she was born. We keep Richard's things in this trunk for safe keeping. David, you can keep that jar of marbles, but I think we will put his other things back in the trunk."

She smiled. "Joan, this was my wedding dress. Do you like it?"

Joan said, "It is very beautiful. Mom showed us her wedding dress too." Kate and Janette nodded agreement.

We packed things away in the trunk and closed it.

Later that evening, Mom and Dad told Johnny and me more about the twins. Dad told us about Rose Mary and how that damnfool doctor got rattled delivering his first set of twins and pulled the umbilical cord off so Rose Mary bled. The doctor transfused Mom's blood to her, but it was the wrong type so it killed Rose Mary, and the lead nurse yelled her head off at him. Dad was upset talking about that. "I had to take that little coffin in the back seat of the car and drive from Anamosa to Audubon with it all by myself for the funeral. The twins are buried together." Then he couldn't talk. I knew where they were buried because we drove there each Memorial Day.

Mom said, "After Richard was killed, we moved to Tom Welch's apartment while we remodeled the house here on the farm. Do you remember that, David?"

"That was where we lived when Johnny was born," I said, knowing I needed to talk about this. Johnny was listening to every word. "Johnny sort of replaced Richard," I said.

"It might look like that to some people," Dad said, "but we wanted another baby. Not for a replacement. Johnny is his own reason for being with us. No body could replace Richard. You probably think of our family as four people. I always think of six."

After awhile Mom said, "It was hard for me to have another baby because I was almost too old. I was 32. But we had to get out of town. David, when you were little you would sneak out of the

59

house and go hide. Then I would come and find you. You needed to be alone, somehow. You still do, so we moved to the country where you wouldn't get run over. It scares me when Dick Jones comes roaring by in that green Dodge."

Nevertheless, they were never overprotective like they did not forbid me to climb way up in trees. I learned I could never get lost in the Hills. I learned to shoot a Daisy Red Rider B.B. gun. It was a sin to kill a goldfinch but not a sparrow or starling. I learned how to ride a bike, but when I crashed it into a patch of nettles they just said I should wash the burning welts with baking soda. I learned if it burned or itched, you washed with baking soda. I learned to put mercurochrome on my own cuts and scrapes. I learned that goose berries turned purple when they were ripe and they were delicious, but the birds got there first. I learned about poison ivy. I learned how to leap from rock to rock barefoot and never get my feet wet. I learned to go barefoot in the summer with callused soles just like Jesus, "who waxed strong in spirit, filled with wisdom: and the grace of God was upon Him . . . and he grew in favor with God and man."

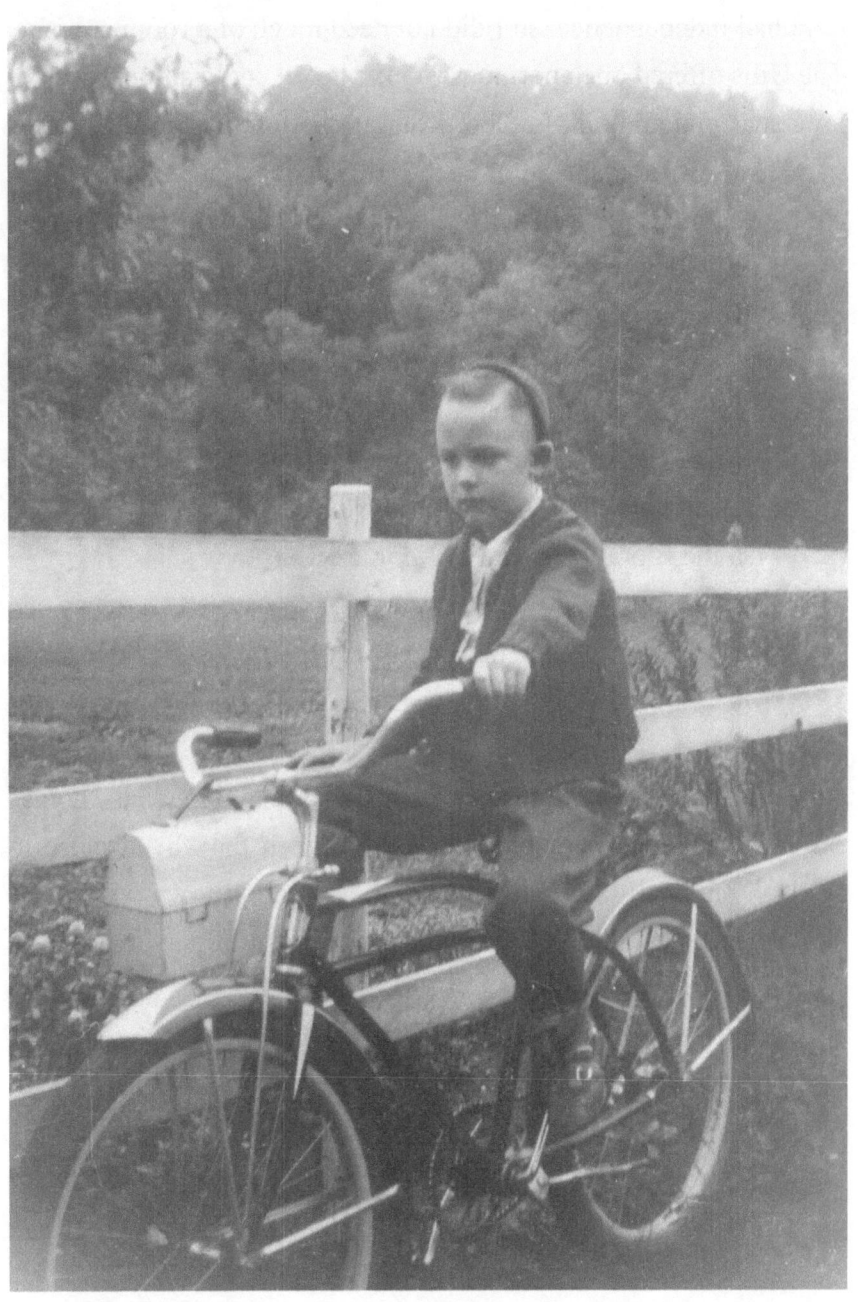

Ready To Roll

I had independence, so I did not need much of a room at home. The Hills offered one enormous room where I could sit on a rock or on a coal pile and talk to God. I buried the marbles and Richard's sacred stuff in a Mason jar up in the Hills under a big oak root. I had a huge advantage over the city slicker kids. Did my parents give up too much? Would I give up electricity, telephone, running water, and roads to live on a farm?

> There are children lucky from dawn till dusk,
> But never a child so lucky!
> For I cut my teeth on "Money Musk"
> In the Bloody Ground of Kentucky!
>
> "The Ballad of William Sycamore"
> Steven Vincent Benét

Best of all, I learned history from Dad. He told me that Thomas Jefferson believed people behaved best when they lived close to the land on small farms. I understood. Moving to town with all its conveniences entailed an enormous curtailment of personal liberty for me.

Shade Tree Mechanic

I was riding my bike in front of the Joneses' house and Old Jim Jones waved me over to him. He was standing next to his work bench. It was inside a lean-to built next to an enormous elm tree in front of their house. Old wheels and broken machinery littered the area, but his tools were neatly put away. Everything smelled of grease.

"You have a shimmy in your front wheel," he said. "Let me see your bike." I got off my bike and let him work on it. "Can't yer dad fix a bicycle wheel shimmy? He's a city slicker." Old Jim did not wait for a reply, but took a wrench and worked on my bike.

While he was working, we heard Dick Jones coming fast. You could hear his loud pipes in his pre-war Dodge. It was green with a steering wheel knob displaying a girl in a bikini. He got out of his car with his lunch bucket. He was young, strong, and sixteen and he had his first car. He wore gray coveralls and he was covered with gypsum dust. He grinned at his dad.

He's been drinking, I thought. *He has a car and spending money now.* Dick Jones never went back to school after he finished the Eighth grade at Holliday Creek School. As soon as he could, he got a job at United States Gypsum. He worked take-off at USG. Dad told me that "take-off" means two workers would take the finished sheets of sheetrock off the assembly line and stack them on a palate.

It was dusty, hard work. Dad said all the mill workers would buy beer when they left US Gypsum for the day. They said it washed the dust out of their throats. Dad said that is why you get an education. Dad also cautioned me to get off the road if I heard Dick Jones coming.

"You drinking again?" Old Jim said. "Smoking too."

Dick walked into the house. He wanted to eat and go to town. Old Jim looked me in the eye. "He goes to town at night with that Norman Smith. They hoot around with girls. He spends all his money on beer and girls. He needs to get out and on his own like Jimmy before he gets into trouble."

Kate walked out the door. She carried trash down to the Creek and dumped it. As it was the spring, the floods would carry it all away. Old Jim always calls it "the damn crick" because it flooded a lot and it threatened the Joneses more than us. Dad would take our trash to town and put it in the garbage can at Carpenter School because he was going there anyway.

Old Jim finished adjusting my wheel. "Try 'er," he said.

I rode off and came back. No shimmy. "Thank you, Mr. Jones," I said.

Old Jim nodded and spit between his shoes, and then he turned to a carburetor clamped in his vise.

Dewey

It was November 1948 and I was in First grade. It was a rainy Tuesday evening, and when Dad got home he took Mom, Johnny, and me to Coalville to vote. They were Republicans and they were going to win.

"At long last we are going to get a Republican in the White House," my dad said. Dewey was supposed to win in 1948, and Dad and Mom had talked about it for weeks. The gravel road was smooth. Dad said the road graders had been out the last couple of weeks because the township was Democratic and they wanted a good voter turnout. Good Republican people like Dad and Mom were voting for Dewey. Rich farmers like Bob Jordison were Republicans. Mill workers were for Truman, but their bosses were for Dewey, Dad said. The teachers at Dad's school were mostly Republicans, but the custodian was a Democrat. "It's a matter of education, you see," Dad said.

We arrived at the school in Coalville. There were lots of cars out front and people with umbrellas. There were farmers with straw hats, bib overalls, and denim jackets. There were lots of mill hands with gray coveralls, and they were all covered with white gypsum dust. Dad wore a suit and a yellow bow tie. He also had a fedora. Dad was a Republican.

We saw Jack Gorelle out in front. He was handing out Truman buttons. He had a brand new pin-striped train-engineer-style cap.

As Dad walked by him, Dad said, "Good evening," and nodded politely.

"Good evening," said Jack Gorelle. "It's a hot time in the old town tonight for sure." He grinned. Then he turned quickly and gave a button to a man and his wife. "Vote for Harry Truman. He's the working man's president."

Dad and Mom voted. There were lots of people standing in line to vote. We voted and went home.

Dad sat out in the car most of the evening because the car had a radio and he could hear the news about the election. The batteries for the radio in the house were dead. They were always dead. Dad was very upset that evening when we found out that Truman actually won.

The Cave

We had no basement, but we had the cave. It was for food storage, not tornadoes, because tornadoes never follow valleys. The cave had been dug into the hillside. Its entry was lined with brick and it had a brick façade over the mantle.

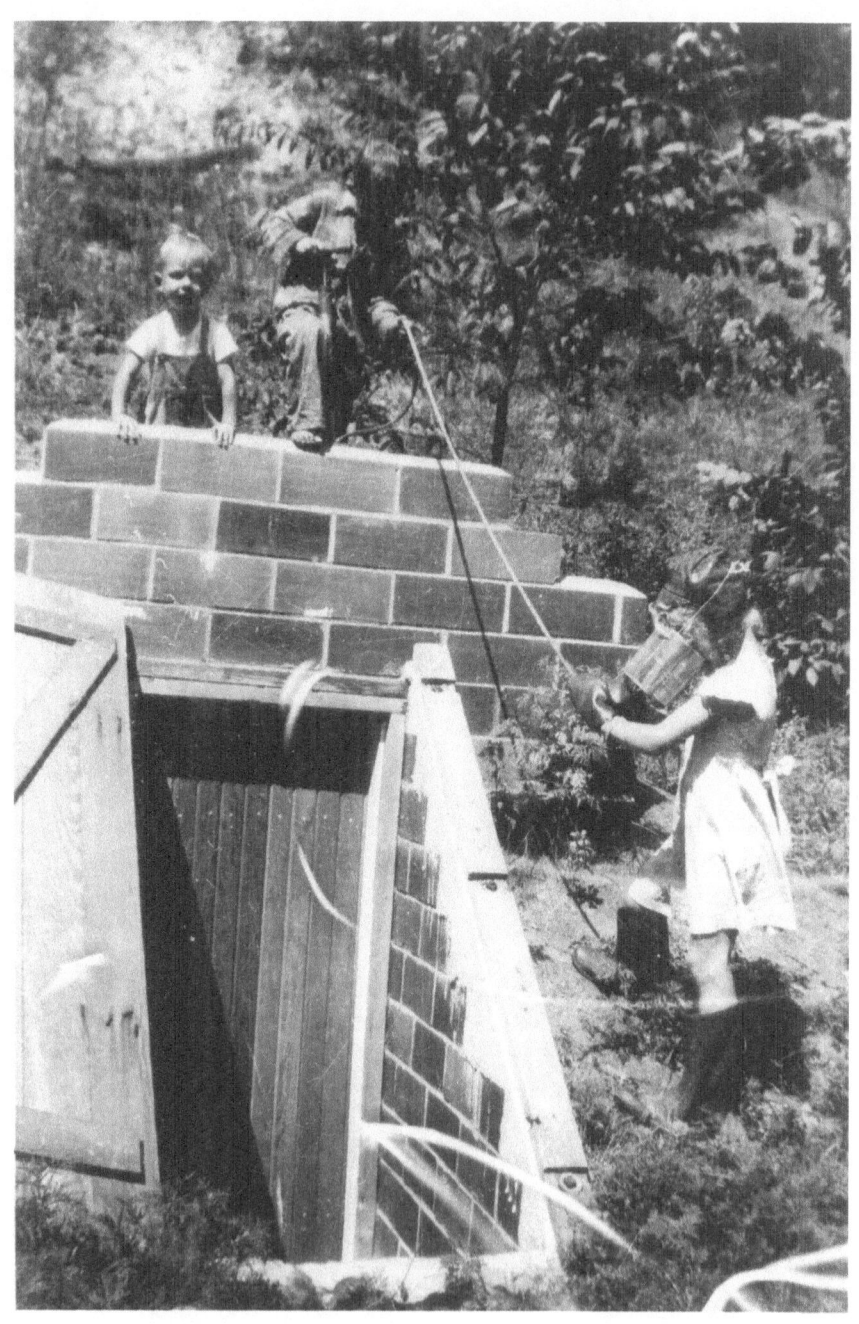

The Cave

One time Mom photographed Janette, Johnny, and me playing Deep Sea Diver around the cave. We had seen a cartoon movie in Fort Dodge about a diver with a long rubber hose going from the ship to the sea floor. The diver had lots of adventures. Janette and I rigged up a piece of garden hose and some sort of bucket for a helmet. Then we played Deep Sea Diver.

The photo shows an outer door like a garage door, but it had an inner door as well, like a door to a room. To insulate the cave in winter, Dad would set bales of straw between these doors. The cave never froze in winter. It was cool and dry in summer. To make the cave, someone had dug a trench back about ten or twelve feet into the side of the hill. It was eight feet wide and at the back of the cut it was about five feet high. Then someone laid bricks upon bricks curving overhead to where they met, supporting one another. All the dirt was piled back on top of the cave and grass grew on the dirt. When I thought about it, it was a wonder nobody got conked by a falling brick. Rain never came in. I knew this was something like how pioneers started on the prairie.

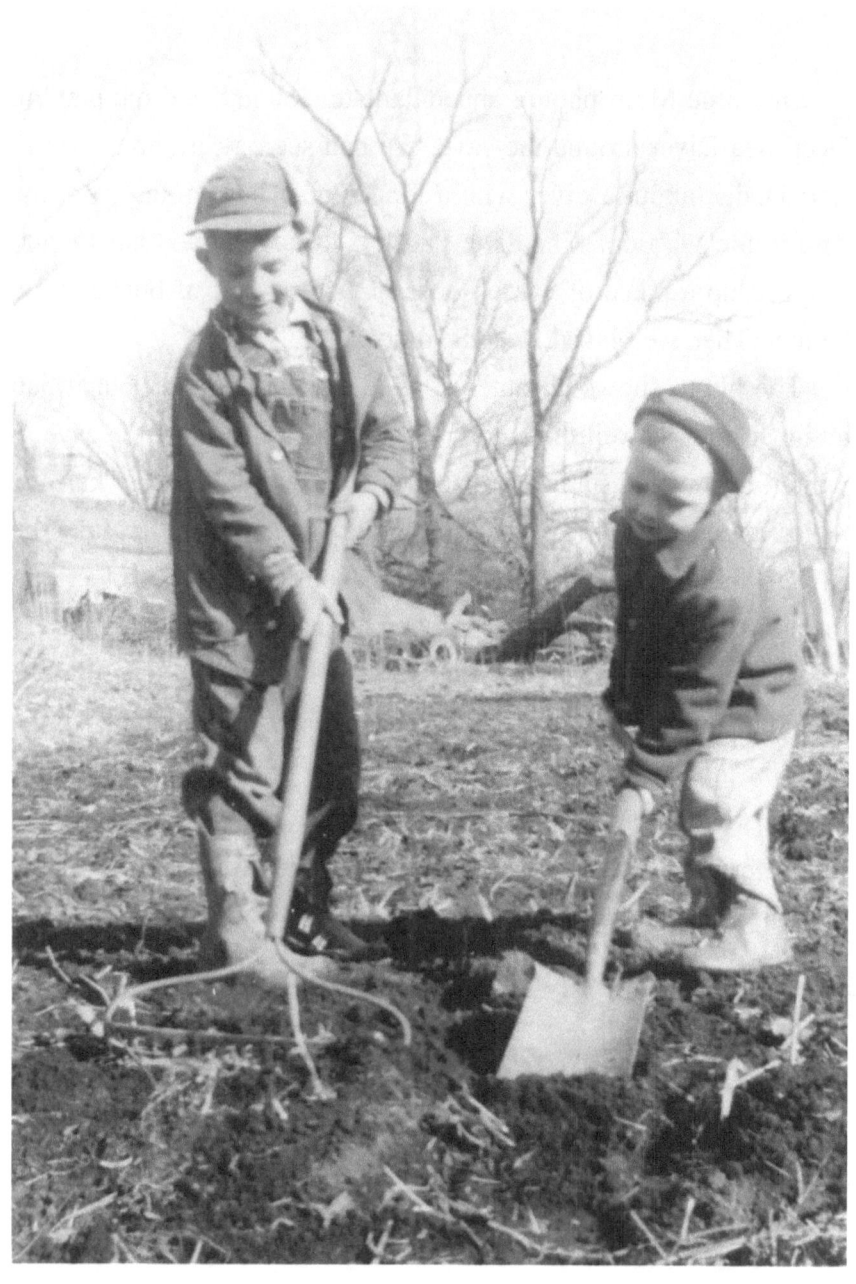

The Gardeners

We piled baskets upon baskets in there filled with potatoes, onions, beets, and squash from our garden. Mom canned often using her new pressure cooker. We stored the jars in the cave. We stored walnuts in there, too. Cracking walnuts and digging nut meats out with a nut pick was tedious work, but if we wanted brownies or cookies . . . Thankfully, Old Jim had a corn sheller that would strip walnut hulls from the actual nut.

Johnny and I often had to go into the cave and thumb the white sprouts off the potatoes to keep them from going to seed. We fed the sprouts to our chickens. Sometimes I would close the door on Johnny and pretend I was the ghost.

Snowed In

A Stormy Winter Night

The storm wind makes the trees all groan.
I hear them twist and pop and moan,
And it is night and I'm alone.
But it is cozy in my bed.
I pull the covers up over my head.
The storm will keep on with its roaring,
But Dad's nearby and he is snoring.

David Wright
Northwest Iowa poetry contest
January, 1950

On one Sunday, after church we went to The Red Arrow, the one grocery in Fort Dodge open on Sunday. It was starting to snow, and a big storm was on its way. Schools were never closed in Fort Dodge. Country schools were a different matter. We had done our usual shopping the day before, but we needed extras because Dad would be staying in town with teacher friends. Either that or he would stay in a hotel. It happened every year. There was no panic, but while we drove home it started to snow and the wind hit us hard. I was very happy because if we were snowed in it meant no school. We bought extra batteries for the radio and white gas for the Coleman gas lanterns. This was before we got electricity or telephone.

Back at home, we unloaded the car while Dad packed. He did not eat. He kissed Mom. Then he looked at me and said, "I've got to go. I am not going to worry, because you are the man of the family now and you can do the jobs I normally do while I am gone. Take care of your mom and Johnny." He drove off into a swirling snowstorm. We all stood silently together as he disappeared up the lane.

The wind roared, and we watched the storm come on. The Jones girls knocked and came in. They were playing in the snow, so Johnny and I went out with them and played in the snow. We yelled and whooped and the wind grew louder. Then we all went inside.

Mom decided we should make soup. Janette and I went out to the cave with the flashlight and got onions, carrots, and potatoes. They were in baskets from our garden. We had plenty of food. Meantime Mom, Joan, and Kate were simmering beef shanks and bay leaf in a pot. It smelled good. We peeled things and put them in the pot. The storm was blinding. It was not piling up on fence posts but blowing into drifts. The road would be shut in an hour.

The smell of soup reassured us. Mom got out a book of poems. We read "Snowbound" that starts, "The sun that brief December day rose cheerless over hills of gray." She played the piano. I played a couple of songs. The Jones girls tried too, but they had pretty much given up on piano. Johnny beat a toy drum to keep time. It was getting dark, so the Jones girls ate and took some soup home. It soon got dark and we tried to get the news but reception was bad. Mom pumped up the gas lanterns and read a magazine, so I read a story to Johnny and we went to bed.

I knew that the next day I would have to carry the honey bucket from our indoor chemical toilet out to the outhouse and empty it. I was also expected to get water from the spring. That was not fun to think about, but it was okay because there would be no school. I thought about fun things to do the next day while I dozed off. We would probably go sliding. When the lane drifted shut it made a gorgeous toboggan run. The wind outside did not scare me. It made me feel warm under the blankets. Johnny climbed the ladder to my upper bunk and crawled in with me. He said he was cold. We slept.

The Cardinal

The Cardinal Poem

The red bird did alight
Upon a branch one winter twilight.
It pecked orange berries frozen tight.
Red and black against all white.
It flew into the coming night.
To show I wrote about this sight
I'll sign below. I'm

David Wright
2012

The December sun was sinking fast, but David knew his way in the woods. He was home from school and anxious to get back in the Hills after the snow of the previous night. After a snowfall everything is new. It was not very cold. He often hunted with his BB gun right after he got home. He stalked sparrows—very seldom getting close enough for a shot. When he killed them near the house and barn, he fed them to the cats, but today he was in the Hills, and he became a big game hunter stalking a snow leopard in Siberia. He heard a show about that on the radio. He loved the word "stalking."

Dad told him about Siberia when he asked. Dad knew everything like that, but Dad did not go into the Hills much. He never hunted. This afternoon David had followed tracks he was sure were bobcat. He had followed them up the Slope. You could tell bobcat from raccoon and fox. There were rabbit prints everywhere. They were food for bobcats.

A bobcat print had four toes like four circles with a big blob behind. It was like a cat's print, but bigger. Granddad Bryan had taught him that. Granddad Bryan chewed and smoked, and he lived on a farm, too, with Grammy. He told great stories about fishing and how his father was in the Civil War, and he had taught David that fox prints are always one exactly behind the other. Raccoon prints looked like tiny hand prints. Raccoons were never in the Hills, though. Old Jim said coons lived down by the crick. They were always pawing through his garbage.

These were bobcat tracks, for sure, but they seemed bigger than most. Maybe they were lynx tracks, he thought. No. Nobody had ever seen a lynx in the Hills, but maybe these were Siberian Tiger or Snow Leopard tracks. The thought brought a shudder. A male cardinal perched on a branch of a berry bush a few feet away; its tufted head and black "V" around its eyes and breast contrasted to the gray-red of its wings and back. It pecked at orange berries among the brown leaves, looking around, nervous.

White, untouched snow made a backdrop with absolute silence; black trunks of trees framing the picture. The cardinal flew. He thought about that and headed down the hill and home. It was so hard to keep a beautiful thing. He would never shoot a cardinal. That was a rule you learned from the Hills themselves when they spoke to you.

Shepherds

It was March and the forty ewes we had were getting ready to deliver lambs, and we all knew it. Most of the snow was gone, but the weather forecast said possible snow. Clouds were rolling in, but it was Saturday night and it was easy for Mom and Dad to think the storm would pass over, so they paid Joan Jones to babysit Johnny and me. They drove to Des Moines to watch the musical *Showboat*. They loved shows, and they figured the storm would pass over, but it didn't.

By midnight the storm was at full force, so when they got home they went out for the sheep, although still dressed for the show. While they did this, Joan, John, and I were asleep on the couch. My parents had just one flashlight and a kerosene lantern between them. They found the flock a half mile away in the Hills, and what a sight! Ewes were in labor everywhere. They were bleating and humped in labor. Dad and Mom would grab a lamb and help pull it out. Then they would go to another and do the same thing. They were not shepherds or veterinarians so they worked in panic.

By dawn, many lambs and ewes were dead. My parents had moved what was left of the herd into the barn. It is hard to move sheep. Twin lambs were left outside to die alongside their dead mother near the carcasses of other dead sheep. Dad was exhausted, but he summoned enough courage to go back out and bring in the twin lambs. In fact, he brought them in to our house. "Twins" was a big word in our house back then. The two lambs would wake Johnny and me up next morning. Baa.

Our world changed that night.

King David

Lambs need care, so we took them out to the barn. Several ewes had newborn lambs, but none would adopt an orphan. Instead they would butt the lamb as it tried to approach, knocking it down. That was rejection. Mom and Dad kept them in the house for a few days, feeding them with a baby bottle. We let the herd go back out to the Hills, but we kept the orphan lambs in the barn. Johnny and I bottle fed our lambs before and after school. They would butt against the bottle. That is how the lambs butted the ewes' udders. I liked the feel of lambs' wool.

I was sent into the Hills every day to count the herd. Usually they were within a half mile of the house. There were still forty-one sheep. Out of forty ewes and one ram there were still thirty ewes eight lambs with the herd and two in our barn, and a ram. Ten ewes died in the blizzard. For a long time the carcasses stank real bad. They were crawling with maggots, and flies swarmed everywhere. Birds would feast on the maggots. Eventually, there was just wool draped over rib bones. Finally weeds grew up around the carcasses. I would see Old Jim and he would say, "How is the sheep herder?"

Dad read to us about David in the Bible from a book full of Bible stories for children. Dad told me that David means "beloved." David was a shepherd boy and he killed a lion and a bear with a sling. Later he used a sling to kill Goliath. I thought that was okay, but I asked Dad what a sling was. Dad explained it was not a slingshot made with a piece of latex rubber inner tube and a Y-shaped stick. He did not finish explaining, but a few days later he brought home a piece of leather from the shoe shop as well as some leather boot laces. Together we punched holes in the leather rectangle and made a sling. Dad and I tried to teach one another how to throw rocks with a sling. This was different from playing catch.

Dad showed me how to put a rock in the leather cradle. He tried twirling it around his head and finally got the rock to stay in there. He whirled it around his head then let one end of the rawhide go letting the rock fly away. He didn't hit anything. He told me to give it a whirl, as it were, and I did. I learned how to throw a rock that afternoon, and for a couple of weeks I tried to hit things with it. I could throw a rock but I couldn't even hit the barn. I marveled about using a sling to kill the giant Goliath. A sling was much more powerful than a BB gun, I decided.

David became king. King David. Dad also read the story of David and Jonathan to Johnny and me. I learned more about David later in life.

Mom said David wrote psalms. I loved the psalm that started, "The Lord is my shepherd, I shall not want. He maketh me to lie down in green pastures. He leadeth me beside the still waters." Mom told me that David wrote that psalm. I pictured just such a place down by the butternut tree near Holliday Creek.

I spent a lot of time taking care of sheep. Dad gave me a special brush and showed me how to pull cockleburs out of their wool. The sheep would hold perfectly still when I did. I liked the feel of wool. I was supposed to pull up cocklebur bushes, but I never did.

That was about the time when Mom got me to write my first poem. Mom got my poem published in a small Iowa poetry booklet for a contest. I saw my name in print for the first time.

I also learned about Jesus' birth and how the shepherds were *sore and afraid* of the Angel on High. (In our Christmas Program, this angel was portrayed by Joan Jones. I was a shepherd in the program.)

Dad told me that Jesus went out after the lost sheep. I knew about going after stupid lost sheep. If one of the sheep wandered off, I would have to find it and chase it back to the herd. I was not very patient. Sheep need to be led, not chased, I learned. Dad got me to understand that people are like lost sheep sometimes. I said, "You mean kids like Roger Sadler?" Dad said, "Yes. Kids like Roger Sadler. Or when you cut through Oren Gray's place with Janette." Dad taught Sunday school at the First Methodist Church.

Dad taught me Jesus is the good shepherd, and that a shepherd is prepared to die protecting his sheep. He will take on a lion or a bear, for instance. He does not let his sheep die out in the snow. Dad said he had not been a good shepherd that night, and those ten rotting carcasses proved it. I knew he was thinking about Richard. Richard was never very far away from us. The trunk was always there to remind us. I wanted to say something to him about that but I was never able to find the right words at the right time.

The lambs grew strong, and they would follow us around the yard. I wanted to take the lambs to school and show them to the kids and let them feel their soft, oily wool, but Mom didn't let us. She recited and sang the song "Mary Had a Little Lamb." This included the verse that went "It followed them to school one day which was against the rule because it made the children laugh and play to see a lamb at school." I could visualize that! Miss Jordison would have a fit. Jack Gorelle would find out and make trouble, I decided.

That summer we had the sheep sheared. A man came to the farm and sheared them. They looked all yellowish with their wool coat gone. The man who sheared the sheep was strong but very gentle. He said that sheep bones break very easily. You have to be gentle. He had very soft hands. He said it was from the lanolin in the sheep wool.

Dad sold the bundles of wool and told us there would be no profits from the sheep. Dad decided to sell them and take his loss, but not until the lambs were weaned.

The lambs were getting grown, and instead of playing with us as they had before, they started getting rough. The male lambs would butt one another, and that is how they got called rams. One day, in the sheep pen, Johnny's lamb butted him and knocked him down. He butted Johnny again when he tried to stand up. I kicked at it and got Johnny out of there. Johnny was crying bloody murder. He was scared. I told Dad, and a week later we loaded all the sheep in a truck that hauled them off to Gowrie, a town nearby with a slaughterhouse.

A few months later Dad said he had to go to Gowrie for some reason. Johnny said, "Dad, don't go to Gowrie. Lambie went to Gowrie and he never came back!"

Maple Syrup

Up in the mountains, it's lonesome all the time,
(Sof' win' slewin' thu' the sweet-potato vine).
Up in the mountains, it's lonesome for a child,
(Whippoorwills a-callin' when the sap runs wild).
"The Mountain Whippoorwill,"
Stephen Vincent Benét

The Hills had sugar maple trees galore. In the fall they turned a gorgeous red. In the spring, however, Dad bored holes in them and inserted a tin spout in the hole. We hung large tin cans below the spout to catch the sap.

We did not collect maple sap in huge quantities. It was like a big experiment from a book I read about pioneers and how they lived. We collected enough sap to make a few jars of maple syrup. One coffee can of sap would make a couple of tablespoons of maple syrup. We never made sugar.

We tapped a dozen trees very early in spring when there was still snow on the ground. Each day I would go from tree to tree and pour the sap from the tin cans into a bucket and bring it home. Mom would boil it off on the stove to make syrup. The trick was not to scorch it. It was great on pancakes and ice cream.

Riding the Willows

I knew how to play alone. I loved to play bat and ball, but that was at school. I did not want to stay indoors and listen to the radio or read. I did not like to play dolls with Janette or play Getting Married or Tea Party. Often I would talk to my Mom and play with Johnny.

On one particular day, Mom was ironing; thus, talking was a real opportunity. Hunting with my BB gun was an option, but it was too muddy to hunt. Most of the snow had turned to water and ponds were everywhere, among dirty, melting snow drifts. I liked fishing, but it was too early to fish. It was great to have so many choices, but for that day I decided to take Johnny and head for the willows.

It was April, so it was not so cold for Johnny. For my purposes, April was fine for willows because they are still leafless, but thawed out and springy. They are just starting to put on buds. In a couple of weeks Mom would cut fresh pussy willows and put them in vases. In winter willows are brittle with frost and they simply snap off. And in summer willows are full of leaves, sap, and bugs. But April is perfect.

Johnny and I got to the willows, and I showed Johnny how to climb. He was easy to teach. He loved to climb, so I showed him how to stay close to the trunk on the way up and go hand over hand to the top. You always drew your weight in toward the trunk on the way up, but you extended your arms and leaned back to make the willow sway. These willows would not grow much over fifteen feet, and they bent easily, so I coaxed Johnny to the top and got him to walk way out on a limb, but not a limb that was too low down because the willow will bend best at the top. I showed him how I would swing my legs full out and make the willow tree bend down. Then I let go and free fell to the ground and let the willow tree snap back upright. About one tree in three broke so you had to be ready for a hard fall. Fun always has its risks.

Johnny fell hard once, getting the breath knocked out of him, but he was tough and went back up and swung on down again. He loved swinging on willows. I know I broke a rib or two swinging willows. I think I was sore for awhile after nearly breaking my neck riding a willow tree.

It is a pity that we did not have birches in Iowa like Robert Frost wrote about in Vermont, but when I read *Birches* for the first time I thought of riding willows. Dr. Eckley pooh poohed the idea of riding willows when I tried to relate my experience in a seminar for a course called Modern American Poets. I felt like a hick. That was at Drake University. You were not supposed to like Robert Frost and rural themes during The War on Poverty. Instead, we were deferred to more existential poets like Wallace Stevens or T. S. Eliot.

We saw birch trees sixty feet tall when Dad took us to fish in Minnesota, but neither Johnny nor I ever climbed one and rode it all the way to the ground. Some opportunities are lost forever.

Oren Gray and Cutting Through

Oren Gray was as old as the hills. The farm he owned was by the bridge over Holliday Creek, so we passed his place every day on our way to school. He knew all our names and always waved. We would see him riding in the Hills. He could see you from far away. He raised horses, so we liked to think of his place as a ranch. He had a large barn with lots of stalls for horses. Cliff Benson worked for him often. The Benson farm was across the road. Oren Gray also hired Sammy Evans to work around the stables. Sammy's job was to clean stables and feed and water horses. He also took them out for exercise. Oren Gray raised big black Percheron horses and sometimes Shetland ponies. Rich people bought them but he told me Shetland Ponies were especially bred to haul coal out of mines, not just to be cute. Dad said we could not afford a Shetland pony.

Oren Gray purchased hay from the Joneses. Janette and I followed the horse-drawn hay wagon on bikes. We watched them unload a whole wagon load of hay onto a kind of net, and using pulleys, hoist the whole shebang into the haymow. One time I saw someone try to cram an oversize forkful of salad into his mouth and I thought of the hay.

One Sunday morning, Oren Gray's barn caught on fire. He and Cliff Benson fought it, but they needed help. They saw the Harris car coming and got them to stop. Kelly Harris told him they would be glad to come back and help fight the fire after church, but right now they had to remember the Sabbath. God came first. Oren and Cliff got all the horses out, but they lost the barn and a lot of saddles and a priceless harness with silver buckles.

Sometimes Janette and I would cut through Oren Gray's property on our way home from school. We would leave the road on top of the Hill and scramble down the rocky slope and cross the Creek. He would see us cutting through from a long way off, but he told us he didn't mind as long as we did not disturb his horses.

We would cut through in the fall when water in the Creek was low. We knew where there was a huge cottonwood lying across the Creek. But usually we would just leap from rock to rock when the water was low so it was okay if we got our feet wet. In summer we did not need the cottonwood, but in winter we used it unless the Creek was frozen. We would see footprints of raccoon and mink and fox in the snow crossing the cottonwood. Mom and Dad told us never to cut through Oren Gray's farm, especially when the water was high.

One day in March Janette and I were lagging behind Kate walking home and we decided to cut through and surprise her by beating her home. The ice was breaking up and the water was dangerously high. We scrambled down Oren Gray's steep hill and headed for the cottonwood. When we got there we stopped. The water was roaring. Big slabs of ice were banging on the cottonwood. The water was brown and ice chunks were piling up behind the cottonwood. Janette and I were daring one another about who would go first.

Suddenly, Oren Gray emerged on horseback out of the timber. "Don't try it," he said, calmly. "You two are dangerous together." He sent us back up the hill to the road.

Mud

Spring always seemed overdue. The ice goes out with a rush, and it was fascinating to watch the slabs of ice exiting through the Creek. Then ditches fill with water and ice is replaced with mud. The road beds are firm until the frost goes out. After that cars create ruts. The road graders never work on water-logged roads. They would come down the main road later when things are dried out, but they almost never would grade the lane. Dad parked our car at the top of the lane and walked the last half mile home most evenings. Old Jim and Dick Jones parked their cars up there as well. All three agreed if the Creek flooded we would not be cut off, but mainly they did not want to create ruts. Meanwhile, we kids went off to school.

Mud was everywhere. We boys wore four-buckle overshoes with bib overalls tucked into the top. This is how mothers tried to keep lower pant legs from getting clustered with mud. Sometimes we did not buckle up buckle boots, so they gaped wide open. That was showing off and you were taking a chance because clayey mud was so heavy that if you were not careful your foot would pull out of your shoe that was still inside your overshoe. You would step in mud with your sock still on. Then you would have to pull your boot out of the sucking mire with one stockinged foot ankle deep in freezing mud. You had to rescue your overshoe with one hand while hanging on to your lunch bucket with the other. You had to figure out how you were going to get your sock off and get your freezing muddy foot back in your shoe that was still inside your overshoe that should have been buckled but wasn't. You did not have anything dry to sit down on. The other kids laughed until they cried at the sight of you sitting on your own lunch bucket. You realized you could have sold tickets and, somehow, you did not howl or bawl about your predicament, but instead you sort of performed for them and made them laugh all the more because of Easter and the pure silly idea of spring and all.

We tracked mud everywhere. We splashed mud at one another. Then it would rain. Mom mopped the floor every day. We washed clothes only once a week on a scrub board. I had to help. That was why we wore muddy clothes day after day. At school we used sticks and old wooden shingles to scrape mud off our overshoes before they let us set them inside the door. We swept mud with brooms until they became entirely encrusted. Then they were useless. We had no running water to hose things off, because all water was hand pumped. Clods of mud littered the steps to the school. Coats and scarves got splattered. Brown jersey gloves were always wet and nobody had a dry handkerchief, so we used sleeves. At recess we did not put on our overshoes, so we mostly stayed on the sidewalk and watched the girls jumping rope. Jump ropes swishing through a puddle. We boys threw mud balls at one another going home, settling old scores from the Snowball Wars. We washed the mud off our hands in puddles. Water ran in torrents off the Hills. Lakes appeared everywhere. Our yard was a sea. I was glad to get home, but I would be missing a glove. I did not have a back pack, though. Back packs would have broken us.

We were always prepared for a flood. The water seeped into the outhouse pit at home and the water level rose a foot or two. It made a huge stink. Johnny was afraid to look at it because I told him he might fall in.

"Electwicity"

The Jones girls called it "electwicity". It was a foreign word in the Hills, but it was about to become a part of everyone's lives.

My dad was the one largely responsible for bringing electricity to Holliday Creek. Dad learned how to contact the REA—Rural Electrification Agency—in Clarion, Iowa. Dad interviewed officers from the various REA cooperatives and found he needed to create a new cooperative in order to get federal loans to pay contractors to bring electric power lines to farms. He learned part of your electric bill was to pay for the debt. You paid one dollar per month above your utility bill until the debt was paid. After that your electric bill would go down by one dollar per month. A cooperative was formed when fifty families agreed to join the cooperative and start paying for electricity. Dad had a map with every family in the Hills, as we called our rural neighborhood. He appointed himself director of the cooperative and drove door to door to get people to sign up. There were sixty-five families; we needed fifty signatures. He brought all the paperwork to each family door. He carried similar paperwork to bring the telephone. Dad was a Progressive Republican.

Dad pointed out to our neighbors that in 1949 there was huge demand for things like electric lamps, radios, electric fans, and refrigerators. Some people responded, "We did not need all these things before. Now why are they are necessities? Dad replied that electricity is not a faraway idea. Sign the petition and electricity will come.

When Dad circulated the petition to get REA electricity he met every family in the area. He caught the attention of local politicians because Dad gets things done. Dad presented the signed petition to the REA office in Clarion. He had collected more than enough signatures. The paperwork was neatly filled out with Dad as the spokesman for a new cooperative. Within a month the line gang showed up. Robert Frost described it:

> Here come the line-gang pioneering by.
> They throw a forest down less cut than broken.
> They plant dead trees for living, and the dead
> They string together with a living thread . . .

Old Jim Jones had refused to sign the petition for the electricity, but Mom got Maudie to sign for him. Jim found out and he got mad. A month later, however, the Joneses were buying lamps and telephones in town along with the rest. Maudie got what she wanted. We saw them in town. Traffic was snarled as it inched by the appliance store with a TV set on a stand out front.

You can't get TV reception in the Hills, we were told, and TV was for the rich. But Johnny and I ended up with our own radio; Dad bought us a second-hand radio, and we tuned in to radio programs like Tom Mix, Bobby Benson and the B Bar B Riders, The Lone Ranger, Sky King, and Mark Trail. Life was good if you had a radio, but we did not read as much from then on.

Drawing Water

For water we sometimes depended on the Spring up the hill from Old Jim Jones's place. We had a well at our place, and a pump, but the water was polluted. You could wash with it but not drink it. Dad brought two five gallon cans of water home from Carpenter School in town most nights, but sometimes we ran out.

Jim Jones had the best water in the world, and he never charged a cent for it, but you had to walk from his road and climb a stile that crossed the fence and from there you walked up the hill up to the Spring. There was no stream. The water collected inside the round hillside itself like a big natural tit and an ancient steel pipe ran out of it, bringing the water to an imbedded, rusted steel half-barrel water trough. Sometimes it was my job to carry drinking water down the hill from his spring across the stile and back to the road and back to our house. I carried a five-gallon can. Carrying an empty can uphill was easy. Downhill, the can was full, and I had to stop and rest a lot. In school I had seen images of Dutch children with yokes on their shoulders carrying water and I asked Dad if that wasn't a good idea, because of *balance*. Dad said no, looking up from his paper, because this was 1948 and we don't use yokes any more. I remembered seeing pictures of women in Africa in the *National Geographic* carrying water pots on their heads. I could never lift a five gallon water can to the top of my head, I decided. I could never carry ten gallons of water. I got up to the Spring and there was Old Jim with a rake in his hand. He was clearing out his spring.

"You are going to have to wait, David, I've stirred up the water. I am raking out the leaves, but you can tip the water can and hold it down while it fills up from the pipe, but don't try to scoop water out of the water trough sure enough." I did what he said.

"I'll tip the can and let it fill," I said. I placed the can on its side mostly floating with the high side right under the rusty pipe. Water ran out as always and began to fill the pail.

"I thought your dad brought water from town," Old Jim said.

"He does, Mr. Jones, but we ran out." Old Jim said not a thing, but he nodded and watched the water from his pipe flow in. The lower end of the can was sinking so I did not have to force it on down in the water.

"David, you just dipped your pail into the pool and you let in muddy water," he said. "Lordy, lad, didn't your Dad tell you how you can get awful sick from drinking muddy water?" He yanked the pail from my hands and dumped the water out. Then he held the can up to the pipe, rinsed it, and it started to fill once again.

"You belong here in these hills, David," he said thoughtfully. "I'm sad about that. You understand the Hills, and belong in them, but you and your family will move out of here and go on. Move to Fort Dodge. Your dad is a well respected, educated man, but he does not belong here. I belong here in these hills. I belong to them." He nodded to me and I took the pail.

"You know I inherited this place from my dad. Dad's family worked in the coal mines around here before that. My brother died in a mine cave-in. Our bones lie about here. Do you know about the coal mines?"

"Yes sir," I said. "I heard a little from what people like Seth Croonquist say. They tell me things. There are old mines all over these hills," I continued. "They mined coal before they mined gypsum. Janette and I see that. There are coal piles, broken machinery, and shovels up in the hills. Lots of tunnels. I know about those things." *He did not know what he did not know*, I thought.

Old Jim nodded. "My dad was foreman of most of these mines before the war." I knew by then that the war he spoke about meant World War I. Miss Jordison told us the difference in school. My parents talked about World War Two, but that was called The War. Old Jim continued, "I remember Dad. He was strong as hell, but Sundays he used to play with us kids. He got our farm from the Company when it went broke."

Old Jim knew that I knew about the ancient tunnels and forbidden mine entrances. I think he knew about the Shack. Sometimes Janette and I would go inching our way back into the abandoned tunnels, but bats flew out and we got scared and ran away. We would make up stories about trolls and other creatures we encountered back in the mines. We scared one another.

Old Jim continued. "The old mines are here and the hills are here and this is where I want to be." The water can had sunk enough to where I did not have to hold it in place. It commenced to fill and sink.

"I'm a mechanic at US Gypsum," he continued. "But I own eighty acres of bottom land and good pasture and some cows and a spring. I know you think education is important and for sure your parents do, but Jesus Christ, boy, things like drinking water hauled from town, and roads and coal mines and gypsum mills and money and electwicity and education will play out on you. Like the coal mines played out on my dad and my brother. The land. The Hills. Those things last on and on. Like that water coming out of that pipe. It runs on forever, Jesus Christ."

He walked away quickly while I lifted the pail out of the spring. It was very heavy and I was glad nobody was going to set it on my head. Old Jim blew his nose with one finger against a nostril. Then he blew the other nostril and wiped his nose with his red bandanna. He went to the cow pen and brought out the cow and the little calf to drink. I saw them drink water that was probably a little cloudy. I put the lid on the water can and started down the hill to the stile. I had to rest a few times before I crossed the stile because the can was heavy and there was no balance. I had to carry it between my knees. I looked back and noticed how perfect Old Jim's Hill looked just then.

Coalmining in
Webster County
(Part Two)

By Roger Natte

The Holliday Creek-Coalville District

At least twelve smaller companies mined [in the Holliday Creek area] off and on between 1888 and 1940. The dominance of mining in the economy of Pleasant Valley Township, which included Coalville and Holliday Creek, can be seen by the fact that the great majority of men in the township were miners. In 1876 sixty-three percent of the men between twenty-one and forty-five were miners, and in 1880 the percentage had risen to eighty. A surprising number of African-Americans were included among them. Assessor's books indicate that fourteen of the miners in the twenty-one to forty-five year age groups were black, about ten percent of the total. Mining continued sporadically in the district through the entire mining period. The last two commercial mines appear to have been operated by Harlan Rogers and Billy McEwen and both closed about 1936. The Rogers mine was located just to the east of Carbon or Gypsum and employed five men. McEwen's mine was located at the southeast edge of Coalville. McEwen's mine was closed shortly after he,

William (Billy) McEwen, was killed when the roof collapsed on him in 1936.

Although the mines were primarily along Holliday Creek, the town developed at Coalville, two miles west, because it was the end of the stub railroad line from which tracks were run to each of the mines. In the 1880s Coalville had a population of nearly seven hundred . . . Most of the population in some way was associated with the mines. In 1884 the town had three saloons, two general stores, a telephone company and all of the small businesses which might be associated with any mining community. The other town in the district was Carbon or Carbon Junction. It developed at the junction of the Illinois Central Railroad and the tramway/railroad from the Coalville and Holliday Creek mines as the transfer point for coal. It did have a store, a post office, and it claimed a short-lived newspaper. It also had all of the equipment and structures needed for the interchange of cars and the storage of coal. In 1903 the Chicago Great Western acquired the Mason City and Fort Dodge Railroad, which included the Carbon-Coalville stub, and in 1915 that three-mile stub was abandoned. The name of the town Carbon was changed to Gypsum, indicating the loss of the importance of coal to the area and the increased importance of the new mineral. By World War I it had declined to thirty houses and in the forties the last of these was torn down. Neither Gypsum nor Carbon exists today.

The remnant of the mining boom town Kalo is located in [the] picturesque wooded valley of the Des Moines River seven miles southeast of Fort Dodge. The second district to be opened was the Kalo-Otho district and [it] was also highly productive and long lasting. It was distinguished by a coal seam running from five to six feet thick. The first coal to be dug there was mined by George D.

Hart after whom Hart's Ford, a shallow crossing of the Des Moines was named. Later Hart's Ford was renamed Kalo by the railroad executives . . .

Coal Mining Towns

Coal mining towns tended to take on a distinct character. Most were characterized by a rough life style associated with hard working and hard drinking men; often single, transient and often unemployed many days of the year. The Fort Dodge Messenger on November 29, 1878, ran an article on Coalville. "We heard something today about some bloody noses and bruised eyes at the saloon yesterday. It is something that some may think that we should refrain from speaking of but when things get to be so degrading to our town as this it is time someone had something to say. The idea of having regular bulldog fights every night of the week with Sunday well put in is getting too disgusting for us to refuse to speak." The reporter offered a solution to the problem. "If our honorable saloon keeper cannot get along without having such a damning hole he had better shut up his saloon and rely on charitable institutions and reflect on his past life and ask himself, 'Where shall I spend my eternity?'" Apparently his warnings did little good. In 1885 Coalville sported three saloons, centers of low life and considered unsafe to be around after dark. Other coal towns experienced the same difficulties. The population of mining towns was a mixed lot. Some were transients who might be employed for a season or two and then move on to new areas and new opportunities. Many were young single men with no roots or ties. Still others were area farmers who worked in the mines only during the winter when their farm work was light and the market for coal was strong. Miners' wages were seen as a way to supplement farm income.

Going Fishing

David let go of the #10 hook and swung his line and corn-cob bobber from his hand to the middle of the crick. His cane pole balanced in his hand. Beside him were a pail, a knife, and a coffee can with dough in it. He and Johnny had made the dough at home. They had cooked flour, water, and salt and made a rubbery paste. Immediately David saw his bobber begin to dance, but he knew not to jerk. Minnows always found the dough ball right away and made it dance. David knew that if the dough is bread-like or soupy, minnows will take it right off the hook. Johnny sat beside him. Teaching Johnny to fish was getting easier. They were brothers fishing. David liked teaching.

Johnny's bobber bounced and bounced, but David said, "There is a big one down there, but he hasn't decided to take it yet. Don't pull up because it's just minnows making the bobber move." Johnny did not say anything. He watched the bobber. Zing! The bobber went down, and Johnny pulled his cane pole up, setting the hook. The pole bent at the end. Johnny stood up and lifted it, and a six-inch chub came wriggling out of the water.

"Big one. Swing him in," David said, and Johnny swung the chub in to the bank. David caught it dangling midair and unhooked it.

"Deedee!" Johnny said loudly, "Did you see that?"

"I saw that. That's three for you and four for me. When we catch another one we will have enough for supper." David dropped the chub in the pail and watched Johnny as he put a dough ball on his own hook. Johnny swung it out with no instructions. "I'm going to clean these," David said. "You catch the last one all by yourself." He started cleaning fish. The sun was low and it showed silver between the green leaves of the Boxelder.

David always smacked the chub on the head with the knife handle if it was still alive. Next he scaled it with the knife blade. Bluegills and walleyes in Minnesota lakes required a scaler because they had large scales, and it took a heavy smack on the head to stun one, but Holliday Creek usually had only chubs whose scales were tiny, and a knife blade would do. Next he took the head off and ran the knife point up the anal opening to split it open, and he gutted it with a quick thumb movement. Then he put the cleaned chub back in the bucket and grabbed another chub. He left the heads and guts on the bank for the raccoons. He left the tails on because he liked to crunch them with his teeth, but his mother considered a fish unclean if it had a tail. Mom would have to cut them off. Mom had showed him how to clean and gut fish; how to roll them in corn meal; how to heat the oil and ease them into the oil without getting scalded. Mom helped him cook. He liked cooking. Chubs were sweet and crisp and crunchy—bones, fins, tails, and all. Soon Johnny caught the eighth chub all by himself! David showed him how to clean it, and let him make mistakes. Then they washed their hands, poured off the bloody water, replacing it with fresh. They headed home. Johnny wanted to carry the pail with eight cleaned and gutted chubs in fresh water as a prize, and David let him. David carried the can of dough and the cane poles. They could eat fish all summer, he thought.

Fishing

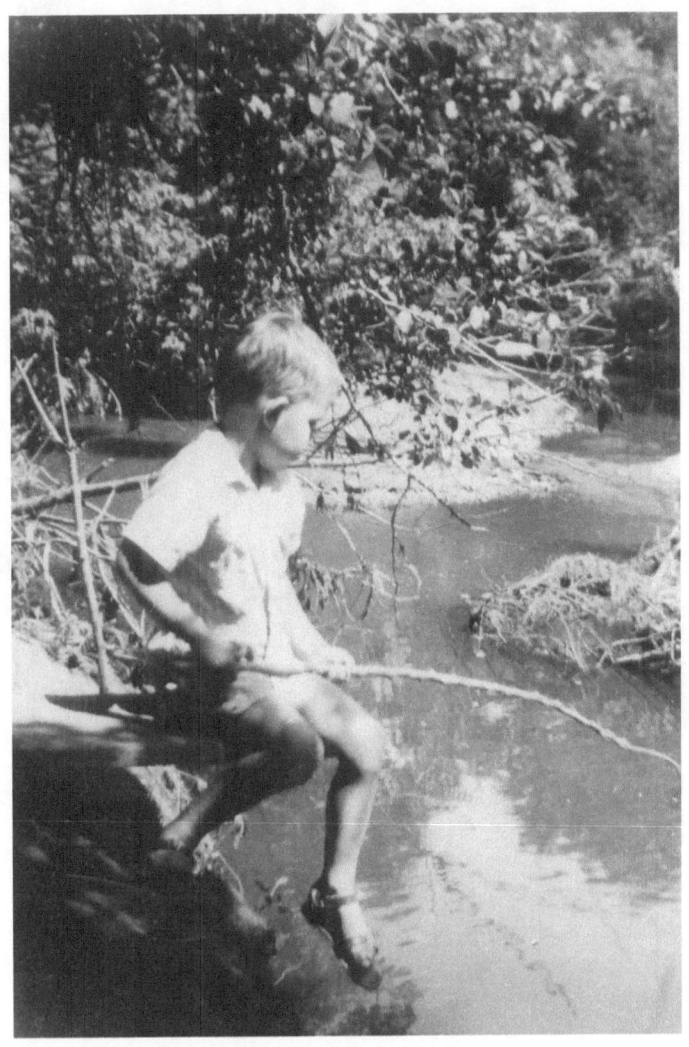

The Fisherman

When I go fishing I always catch a fish.
And then at supper time it ends up in my dish.

David Wright
Northwest Iowa Poetry Contest
1948

Sycamore

Zaccheus he
Did climb the tree
Our Lord to see.
The New England Primer

Nuts to You

It was autumn again and the hills were afire. We gathered nuts in the fall. We knew where—like in spring when morel mushrooms were bursting out of the ground everywhere. City slickers would come out searching, but the Jones girls knew where to find mushrooms, and they always had buckets of them for sale. They got good prices. Jim and Maudie did not raise fools.

Of course, where I lived we had black walnuts and hickory nuts. Best of all were the butternuts—a sweet type of walnut. City people would drive out and buy them from the Jones girls. Old Jim would let his girls spend their own money, but he would not pay for movies or sundaes. Movies cost twelve cents, and they had to get their own money. He did not believe in handouts.

The girls gathered sacks and sacks of walnuts and butternuts. The husks had to come off the nuts or they would rot. City slickers would buy walnuts with the shells on, but not with the soft green husks that covered the shell. The Jones girls scattered the walnuts on the driveway and they hoped car wheels would help grind off the green husks. Peeling husks by hand was a tedious task, and your fingers got raw quickly. Also, if you handled black walnuts your fingers got stained and they stayed stained for weeks.

Old Jim helped to solve this challenge. He would often go to the Sale Barn in Gowrie for bargains. One time, for two dollars he bought an old hand-cranked corn sheller that wouldn't work. He was a master mechanic, and he got the gears unstuck. He found if you adjusted it just right, the corn sheller did a good job of husking hickory nuts, walnuts, and butternuts, leaving the exposed shells in a heap with the husks.

It takes land, labor, capital and entrepreneurship for a business. The land produces a tree with nuts on it. (In this case, the butternut tree was on Oren Gray's land; the nuts were free for the taking.) Labor was the girls who would gather nuts and turn a crank. The sheller was capital. Old Jim was also a labor factor when he reached into the sheller to get the gears unstuck. This entailed *risk*. The sheller, as capital equipment, was also at risk. Old Jim acted as the financier, insisting that the first two dollars' worth of walnuts went to pay him back for buying the sheller in the first place. Maudie also got to keep all the walnuts she wanted as a form of interest payment. There were cookies, fudge, and cakes to be made, with an emphasis on butternuts. The girls were entrepreneurs. Their sign was visible on the road.

One October Sunday, Mom invited the Beamer family to visit our farm and go on a nut-gathering and landscape-viewing expedition. Betty Beamer was in the Fort Dodge Art Club, and she had perked up when Mom's paintings of nature won a prize at the Blandon Memorial Art Gallery. She asked Mom to show her how to choose a scenic spot and start a water color landscape. The Beamers ranked in the Methodist Church. Their oldest son, John, was Kate's age, and the twins Jane and Buddy were in my Sunday school class. I knew that my dead brother and sister, Richard and Rose Mary, were boy and girl twins too, and I longed to know what it would be like to be in a family with twins, but all I had to go by was John Beamer, the older brother of Jane and Buddy. John deliberately stepped on my foot when he got out of the car and got introduced. He did not like me or our farm.

The plan was we would all gather nuts while Mom and Betty sketched.

While we were still at our home, John Beamer wanted to use the bathroom. I showed him to the outhouse and explained that we men always stood unless we had to sit like women. He did not understand. He had never seen an outhouse. Their grandfather was with them. He said it was a good outhouse like when he was a boy. He owned a lumber yard in Fort Dodge, and a sawmill somewhere. Mrs. Beamer's husband, Leland, managed the lumber yard. That was where Dad bought the lumber to build the stile. They were city slickers for sure, and tomorrow everyone at school would ask me about their visit. I would tell Larry Jordison that one of the kids peed on the seat. His aim was terrible.

After they went to the bathroom, they wanted to wash hands. They had never seen anyone ladle water out of a pail to wash in. Mom and Betty Beamer made light of it all, and we walked down the road past the Jones place. We saw their sign advertising hulled walnuts and butternuts.

I was embarrassed and I acted like I did not know them, but that was lost on the Beamers, who enjoyed the hike to the butternut tree down on Oren Gray's land. The grandfather kept commenting about all the tall, straight, walnut trees and hickory trees out our way. He appraised the trees. When we climbed the last rise we could see the Des Moines River, all silver below, with Holliday Creek flowing into it. The butternut tree stood by a quiet pool of the Creek. Its branches grew straight out then down and back up forming a "J" at the end. We did not see any squirrel hunters, so it was safe to go down. Mom unfolded two canvas camp stools and started to sketch while Betty Beamer watched, sketched, and asked questions. The rest of us went down to the butternut tree to gather nuts.

The hillside beyond the river had brilliant puffs of red maple with the yellow of cottonwood, Boxelder, and willow mixed in. The oaks were still green, but the stately elms were yellow, while the sky was a brilliant blue. Brown fields of corn were rimmed with trees. A pair of jays flew by the grandpa, crying, "Thief! Thief!"

We saw Oren Gray and Sammy Evans riding horses, leading a Percheron colt with reins between them. They were training it. They looked up our way, and Oren Gray put his fingers to his hat brim and rode on. He was as old as the hills, and this was his land. He would see everything going on. He had riders.

The Beamer kids wanted to leave because they were reminded a cowboy program was going to be on TV. Someone started whining they had to go to the bathroom. We could go back to our house, we said, but they complained they just couldn't go in an outhouse again. I was embarrassed, as I knew what I would have done in that situation. I would have just slipped off and peed behind a tree and found my way back to the group. They did not know how to do this. I knew they would talk to the other kids the next day in Sunday school about our outhouse and water pail. The Beamer kids whined some more about getting back to town and their new TV. They did not want to miss anything. Their dad gave in to them, saying, "The kids aren't used to, uh, such primitive conditions." He winked at my dad—*he actually winked!* "You know how it is." Of course, we did not have a TV, so we did not know how it was. I looked up at my dad. I was going to find out all about it tomorrow in the Methodist Church.

Dad handed him a sack of butternuts. "Nuts to you," he said, smiled, and winked back.

We walked back up to where Mom was sketching. She had a good start on a picture, but the Beamer kids had to get back to their flush toilet and TV. Mom got tight-lipped. We made our way back home.

On the way, the grandfather saw the Jones girls' hand-painted sign and went up to Joan. He offered to swap a bag of unshelled butternuts for a bag of shelled ones and pay the difference. Old Jim watched the deal unfold from a distance. Joan took the money: two dollars. The story would be all over Holliday Creek School and USG in the morning.

What I would remember most about that day was Dad saying a very quiet "Nuts to you." Kind of a *Nuts Dimmintis*. He dismissed them.

Not long after this, Oren Gray's barn burned. He sold many mature walnut trees to a lumber company in Fort Dodge to get the money to rebuild the barn; the loggers cut walnut and maple trees for a week, but he did not let them cut the butternut tree. They also cut hickory trees to sell to Treloar's Inn; Treloar's made world-famous hickory flavored ribs and beans.

The PTA Meeting

Parent Teacher Association meetings were held in the spring and the fall. Jack Gorelle was up for reelection as the Director.

One evening after dinner, Bob Jordison and his wife came calling at our house. Miss Jordison and Jake Foust were with them. He was not a school board member because he lived on top of the Hill, outside the school district. His father had donated the land for Holliday Creek School ages ago, so his family name was important to the community.

They encouraged Dad to run for School Board Director against Jack Gorelle. Dad didn't want to run, though he knew Jack Gorelle appointed himself to do school maintenance and collected a nice paycheck but seldom worked.

"When my boy died, it took all the fight out of me." Dad said. Mom was quiet, although she wanted him to run. Bob Jordison said he appreciated their grief but he pointed out that Dad should get a lot of support because he had circulated the petition to get the electricity. He pointed out that Dad was a college graduate with an administrative credential. Dad was a Progressive Republican, everyone knew. He wore a white shirt and tie every day and wore steel-rimmed glasses like Teddy Roosevelt, whereas farmers and mill workers wore denim.

Dad had a responsibility to serve his community. "That is the basis of democracy," Bob said. He was right, of course, and Dad filled out the appropriate forms in order to run.

In those days the kids went to the PTA meeting along with the parents. It was early October, and we were allowed to play outside while the business meeting was held inside the school.

For us kids it was the most wonderful chaos of all. We were not only allowed to play unsupervised, but in the dark as well. Some of the older kids were supposed to supervise us, but they could not be everywhere, so it was a perfect setting for the most wonderful mischief. We played hide and seek in the dark. No rules. We played Run Sheep Run. No rules. We played Pom Pom Pullaway. Over behind the tree, Marlene Sadler was smoking cigarettes with Donna Smith in the dark. Dick Jones had parked out front, showing off his green pre-war Dodge. And it was dark.

Meanwhile inside, Jack Gorelle had lined up his support against the city slicker. Jack was a Democrat. Stanley Stein, the farmer, nominated Dad. Jake Foust seconded. Dad thought he had the support of J. Clare Robinson, who was County Superintendent of Schools. He knew Dad was a capable school principal in Fort Dodge. He knew Mom had a teaching credential from Iowa State Teacher's College in Cedar Falls. But J. Clare Robinson was a Truman Democrat and he sided with Jack Gorelle during the meeting, endorsing him as "a champion of education for the working class family." Dad was defeated 35-28.

On the way home, Dad and Mom were angry. They felt betrayed. They talked about moving to Fort Dodge. Johnny was asleep in the back seat, so he did not see me cry.

The Flood

Cumulus nimbus clouds look like ice cream, but they bring storms. Dad and I were reading a library book together about weather, and we talked about it during breakfast. Dad always made coffee for me, and we talked about news before I went to school. We looked at a photo in the book. Then he showed me a photo from the *Des Moines Register*. The photo he showed me had a caption that said a Missouri thunderhead went up 48,000 feet, but we did not read about the damage it did. This was science. Dad got me to calculate, mentally, how high 48,000 feet was. I had to go inside my mind and do the math. The process was getting easier. He taught me to "round off."

Well, 48,000 feet is about 50,000 feet. A mile is about 5,000 feet. A little more. Ten miles high; subtract, maybe, one: gives you nine. I am a terrific "rounder off-er" today. The cloud was a huge pile of ice cream nine miles high, I concluded. We laughed at my round-off. We decided at least it had lots of ice, sleet, and hail in it. We were not thinking of damage when he drove off to school, but a storm was on its way and it would impact people.

Sammy

That morning I stopped at the bridge and looked down at Holliday Creek. It was just about back within its banks. A week ago it was flooding, when we had all that mud. I looked over at Oren Gray's. Sammy was already working up on the slope from the house and barn. He was pounding down steel fence posts. He saw me coming and yelled at Oren Gray who motioned for him to go. Sammy walked down the lane and met me on the road. He was sweating. "Do you have anything to drink?" he asked. I opened my lunch bucket and handed him my Kool-Aid thermos. He gulped from it and wiped his mouth.

"You are early," he said. We started walking toward school. Sammy said, "The Jones girls are lagging behind you. I can see that. Mr. Gray said to me, 'You keep on working until you see the first of the kids going to school. Then you lay down the sledge and go on to school.' You are the first kid going to school, David, so I was glad to see you."

Sammy was my friend and protector, but I knew he wanted something. He also knew Chester Wilwhite and I would not let others bully his little brother. Protection gets passed on down. Protection is as old as America.

"Mr. Gray has me and Mr. Benson building a temporary corral up there in case there is a flood. Big storm coming up from Missouri. Corral's about done, so he sent me on to school. I could use something to eat."

I opened my lunch box and he wolfed it all down. When we reached Sammy's place we stopped. He went in. A minute later he lugged out his sleepy brother, Lyle.

I supposed everyone in the house was passed out drunk. That is what *They* said on the school ground. "What are we going to do about Lyle?" I asked.

"Lyle is out of that house for right now," Sammy said. He carried little Lyle for a minute and spoke softly to him. Then Lyle perked up and slid down on the ground and wanted to play. He was going to school.

We kept peanut butter and jelly and bread in the school basement, and if someone needed food, it was there. Sammy, Lyle, and I were going to eat that way today. When we got to school, Sammy took Lyle to breakfast.

David

I wanted to tell everybody about what Dad and I had learned together about Cumulus nimbus. It was important to us all right now; besides, another cloud was building up down in Missouri somewhere even as I spoke, soon to move toward Iowa. School had not yet started, and we were out on the school ground. I wanted to persuade Miss Jordison to let me tell about Cumulus nimbus later during Show and Tell, but right then she was surrounded by girls—a storm of girls, I mused, that seemed to bulge up from Missouri sort of dangerous and full of air and ice. Instead of trying to push and barge in front of them with my message of Cumulus nimbus, I joined the others playing cowboy and got tripped by Shorty Harris, who laughed. He got even, boy. We were always trying to "get even" with one another.

The Little Kids

Across the fence, Jake Faust was a happy man, even though he was gazing at the sky again. *They* said he and Eleanor were going to have a baby. *They* concluded someone was "rubber-necking" on the party line. *They* said Eleanor Faust (Miss Jordison) was talking to a doctor. (Like it was a conspiracy.) *They* said she would have twins. *They* said Miss Jordison would never do *it* with Jake Faust. That was too awful. Ronnie Smith said, "She should not be allowed to have a baby. She needs to take care of us. That's unfair to us." Ronnie Smith was always saying "no fair." The year was ending, and Miss Jordison had changed. She had a dreaminess about her, and also some irritability. The girls quickly understood. *They* asked who would teach next year. *They* said my own mom would teach school next year . . .

Eleanor Faust

There stood Miss Jordison, eyeing the line of cumulus clouds even while she was surrounded by little girls, each demanding her attention. Each one poked her with an index finger and said, "Miss Jordison. Miss Jordison." It must have been like getting pecked to death by chickens. I thought, *She cannot control everything. Take care of yourselves.* Then I thought that the world is like a one-room school house where Jack Gorelle was the government, but where was he when you needed him? Miss Jordison probably was remembering that Jack Gorelle had vetoed the idea of getting a telephone to the school. "Unneeded government spending," he had said. The teacher was there, but controlling everything in school is as impossible as controlling a thunderstorm. As teacher, Eleanor Faust saw herself as responsible for everything, nonetheless, and some people thought she did not deserve a private life. She realized some kids are leaders who helped and encouraged others. Some were enforcers who helped keep the rules and protect others. Weak ones needed to feel protected, and they could learn to be protectors themselves—like Sammy, or Jimmy Jordison, or Kate, who slapped Shorty Harris silly when they caught him bullying. Miss Jordison let them do some enforcing without actually saying so. She had concluded gossip and rumor abounded, in a one-room school house along with cowardice, courage, and a lot of herd instinct, but within its walls was the future of America. She rang the hand bell and all went inside. The day had begun.

Jake Faust

Through the window you could see Jake outside, scurrying from one job to the next on the farm. He knew there was going to be a storm. Miss Jordison tried to keep us from watching Jake. He drove the tractor and wagon into the machine shed. He herded hogs into the hog house, and that was hard because the one hog did not want to go in. We got the giggles. He left that hog outside and closed the door. The hog would have to face its fate alone. He herded cows into the barn and shooed the chickens into the chicken house. I thought of Noah and the Ark. Jake had to bring extra water while they were cooped up inside. Jake took the laundry down from the clothesline. Was it still damp? The girls commented about that. Were his hands clean handling the laundry? Jake disconnected the wind mill so the blades spun on free wheel. He was expecting big wind. Miss Jordison threatened to pull down the shades so we would not be looking out at Jake, but she didn't do it.

Larry Jordison

During Show and Tell, Larry Jordison showed us all a photo of a thunderhead in a day-old *Des Moines Register.* I was jealous. I wanted to tell more after Larry showed the picture, but Cumulus nimbus was not a subject anybody wanted to hear about. It was the same old cloud we were watching yesterday *They* said in agreement. Larry did not mention that Cumulus nimbus clouds always come from Missouri. During morning recess we all saw that the clouds puffing up over Missouri were making for us. It was very humid. School went on, but girls who came in from the outhouse were whispering about "the clouds." It got dark when the storm cell approached us. During lunch I made more peanut butter sandwiches with Sammy and Lyle Evans. Then we went out to look at the line of clouds; and we saw a monster with its white top and others beside it had anvil points. Jim Jones had an anvil on his work bench, so I knew that was the name of that part of the cloud formation. The monster cloud had sort of a mountain look to it. Lightning adorned its slopes. Lightning lit up its black interior. I remembered a library book picture of the stupid dinosaurs when they saw that vast comet plummeting down at them. It was on my mind.

It started to sprinkle, and Sammy said nothing, but his little brother was fed and safe under my protection, so Sammy climbed the fence and made a run for Oren Gray's. Marcia Stein went to Miss Jordison and told on him. A bolt of lightning hit the ground near Sammy's home. Everyone saw him run while it thundered and then it commenced to rain. We all knew he was going to lead horses to the corral on higher ground. We were in for a storm, but then, this was Iowa and we would always get storms.

Miss Jordison

Miss Jordison saw her husband, Jake, nailing down shingles on the machine shed roof. Lightning was banging all around. Janette was excited by the noise and said something about the Fourth of July. Dolores started to cry. Back inside, someone said Miss Jordison needed to decide if school was to be dismissed early. There was no telephone at the school, so Miss Jordison could not call homes. She was composed, even though she knew the kids knew she wanted to dismiss school and run home to Jake. She told us we would stay at least until three o'clock. She slapped the yardstick down hard on a desk. She urged the students to work on their lessons even though her eye was on the clock. It was hard concentrating with all that lightning.

Miss Jordison gave up about two o'clock, but she did not dismiss as usual. She went from child to child saying things like, "Sammy ran off to help Oren Gray. David, you take Lyle, and if no one is at his house that can take care of him; then Jimmy Jordison will take him to his house." And, "Larry, you look after Mike. If no one is home at the Sadlers, Marlene, you and Betty will keep things together. Roger has chores to do. Roger, are you listening? If no one is home at the

Benson house, the Bensons should go back up the hill to the Sadlers. Kate, you are in charge of everyone going south." Then she turned to Bruce Pingle, who would evacuate everyone going north. Parents never picked up their kids at school, except for Marsha Stein's mom, who was already waiting outside.

*   *   *

We kids stuck together on the way home. One or two kids had umbrellas, but after the first quarter mile it did not matter. I left my bike at school. A bike was a detriment, a thing to drag along and not ride in a storm. Nobody answered the door at Evanses, and Lyle started to bawl when the Jordisons took him with them to their house. When we dropped off the Sadlers and Bensons, Janette, Kate, and I looked from the bridge at Holliday Creek. The water was way up, and trees and logs were piling up above the bridge. When we got to our lane we could see the whole floodplain.

Dad got home. He parked up on the Hill and he had two full water cans with him. He had on a good raincoat. He wore a white shirt, a suit, a yellow bow tie and a fedora. Old Jim and Dick Jones arrived at the same time. They walked with him. They wore gray company uniforms, but in the face of a storm all three were equals. They talked. The Joneses were closer to the Creek, so they were in for it. Dad invited them to stay with us. Old Jim said no thanks. "Keep the latch string out, though," he said, and grinned. He shook his head and spit.

Mom had dinner ready. Later, a huge lightning strike knocked out the lights and telephone. We still had white gas and lanterns, and Mom had already filled them. Dad and Mom had already moved the trunk out of the garage to the cave. The cave was a good four feet higher than the house. Water was well over the road and running through the garage. The water reached the barn next, and they moved stuff into the hay loft. We were glad we did not have livestock. Then Dad took me, Mom, and Johnny with umbrellas and the flashlight to the water's edge. We looked through the dark at the rising waters. Johnny was old enough to see the flood. It was drizzling.

"The damage is done." Dad said. "Just how high the Creek rises will be known tomorrow. I think we are okay." The rain eased off and we went to bed. Dad snored so loud it woke me up, but I reasoned if he was sleeping we were all right, so I slept. Then it cut loose during the night. Thunder is exciting and I enjoyed it, but Johnny crawled in with me. It poured all night. It rained eleven inches, give or take.

Dad

Dawn was golden. The Cloud moved off. Dad was golden, even though Creek was halfway across the yard and rising. I talked with him about Cumulus nimbus during breakfast. We drank coffee. Johnny tried coffee and liked it. Dad knew there was more to our lives than Cumulus nimbus. He loved his boys and announced to them he was being promoted in the Fort Dodge School District. He had his mind on that and seemed not to notice even when Dick Jones and Norman Smith went floating by our house in the flood water on an uprooted tree trunk. They eventually let go of it and swam off before the torrent roiled at the bend in the Creek, and they waded back up to our place. They took coffee and sandwiches and talked.

Dick Jones

"Our barn is not gone," Dick Jones said, "but the crick is running through it two feet deep, and we could see the same with our garage. Dad moved the cow and calf up by the spring last night. We put the mechanic machinery in the truck and parked it up along the road." Dick said that the house was not safe for the time being because even though it was up on stilts, the water was underneath the house.

Dick said, "Dad said to all of us, 'It is going to be a sorry mess and a lot of work to straighten this out, but you might as well enjoy the flood. Just don't get hung up on a barbed wire fence and drown.'" Dick and Norman waded back into Holliday Creek with its snakes, raccoons on floating trees, and muddy, icy water. There were lots of logs to ride.

The Wright Family

Johnny and I played in the cold water as it rose. After stirring you up, the floodwaters became a transfixing thing. The flood kind of lulled you even while you were being drowned. A numbness set in. By afternoon the water came up to the second step of our porch. Dad says, "We gotta sell." Then the water went down, leaving a silt pile in our yard to punctuate his words.

The earth solidified so we could use the roads and the farmers could get out in the fields. I was hoping Dad would remember how we came through the mud time a couple weeks back and figure weather would work itself out like that, but he didn't see it that way.

Conflagration

It was more than spring. Spring means an end to snow and a season of mud, howling winds, and heavy rains with the prospect of floods and a soft a dash of pussy willows down by the Creek thrown in. This particular morning, a Saturday, was not an ordinary spring day. We needed water, so Mom sent Johnny and me to the spring. We took two buckets down past the Joneses' place.

The Joneses saw us climbing the stile, of course. Johnny and I went up to the spring and drew the water. I always hated being sent for water, and I would always complain that town kids had running water and did not have to carry two heavy buckets, and that I wished I was a town kid Mom would make me go fetch water anyway. I was always surprised that it was such a pleasure getting water out of that spring once I got there.

I remembered that time a year earlier with Old Jim talking to me about the hills and all. I remembered how we had cleaned out the well together. He had said, "You belong here in these hills, David, but you will not say so. I'm sad about that. You understand the Hills, and belong here, though, but you and your family will move out of here and go on. Move to Fort Dodge."

I stood and looked at that the water flowing forever out of that rusty old pipe. I looked down the hill to the Jones house.

Johnny wanted to carry a bucket on our way back, so I let him. He got tired carrying soon, but not as quick as you might think. He was getting tougher. When I picked up the bucket from him I said, "I can beat you to the stile running with both of these buckets."

"Go," he yelled, and we ran. He got to the stile a good forty feet ahead of me. I knew he would win, but it was fun to watch Johnny run.

"I guess you won that time," I said. Johnny grinned. We climbed over the stile. Then we were at the Joneses' porch. I set down the water cans. Maudie Jones came to the door with Kate, Joan, and Janette behind her. "Hauling water for mom and dad on a Saturday morning, are you? It must be nice to be alone with your man on a Saturday morning with no kids," she said.

"Yes'm," I said. I had never said "Yes'm" in my life, but I had heard it in some movie when the boy wanted to show respect to an older woman.

"Yes'm?" Maudie said. "I don't remember you saying that before, David."

"I heard someone say it in a movie," I replied, "and I thought I would say it."

Janette and Kate started acting out a parody of my play acting, saying, "Yes'm," but Maudie shushed them. "I think your mother has taught you well," she said.

"Janette," I said to Janette. She looked over at me. She had a pajama thing over her but her hair was golden and shining and that was because Maudie Jones had the most beautiful hair of anyone and she taught her girls how to use the brush. Janette was holding shoes in her hand. "I have a new Tom Mix telescope I got with three box tops and seventy-five cents in coin," I said. "I want to try it out." I was nine.

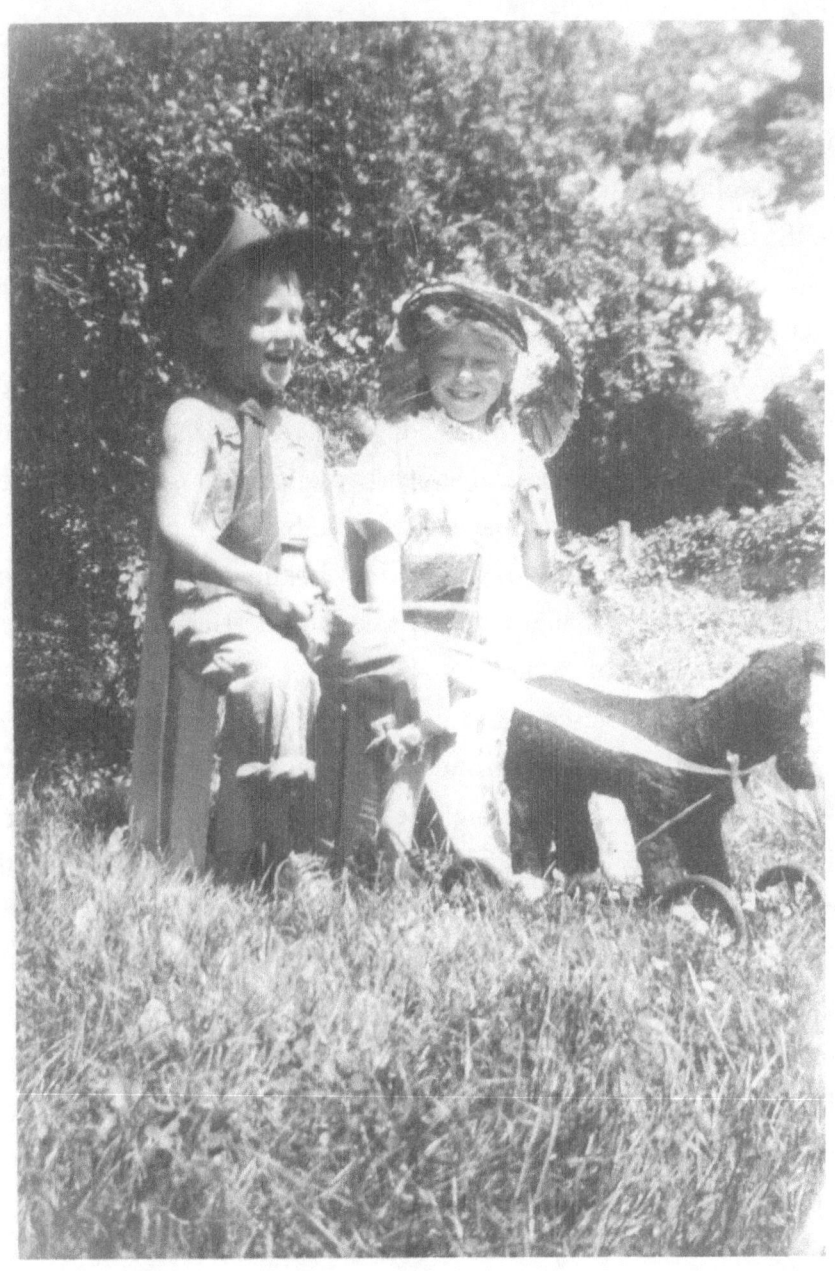

Buggy Ride

"Sure," Janette said. So thirty minutes later I was back on her doorstep. Johnny was at home with Mom and Dad. I had the telescope in my hand and Janette was dressed.

We climbed the stile and went up near the spring. We went up to the top of the hill and turned south toward the Des Moines River and we crawled under the fence onto Oren Gray's land. We both had overshoes and jackets. I had the telescope and I had brought a sandwich (cut in two) in my lunch bucket along with two hard boiled eggs and some salt. I had a thermos of Kool-Aid. Janette had brought apples. Also, he had stolen two cigarettes from Dick who was still asleep. She had matches as well, but she did not show me the cigarettes until she coaxed me into building her a fire on that hilltop looking over the butternut tree and the Des Moines River. There was plenty of wood lying about.

We took the telescope and watched the river. We saw the water was high and muddy brown, but there was no longer any ice. The ice went roaring out weeks before. We agreed not to go near the river. Instead, we took turns looking at the hillside. The telescope slipped out of focus but we saw two fox on the hillside across the valley. Then we saw what they were doing, and we talked about it. I got embarrassed but I changed the subject because we saw Oren Gray on horseback. He was riding toward the foxes, but he stopped and looked our way. The foxes ran away. He looked toward us a long time. We looked back at him through the telescope. We decided he could not see us.

Janette wanted to play Getting Married, and I gave in. It made me feel funny. She coaxed me into it like I did when I tried to coax Jerry Smith into urinating onto the electric fence. He didn't fall for my trick, and so I did not want to get undressed or anything when we played Getting Married, but we ate sandwiches and apples and boiled eggs. We were playing banquet. Then we drank Kool-Aid champagne and smoked the cigarettes.

We were always trying to smoke leaves and corn silks, but stolen cigarettes made us silly, and dizzy and half sick. I wanted to throw up, and lie on the earth looking at the blue sky whirl overhead with the white cloud looking like . . . like smoke rising from the campfire. We jumped to our feet, and the fire was running uphill toward the pasture. There were cattle in the pasture on top of the hill. That was Bob Jordison's place, and we knew we had to stop it. We knew enough from the Western movies that cattle would run off a cliff to avoid a range fire. We knew we had to get in front of the fire and turn it back. We ran ahead of the fire and we grabbed branches and tried to beat the fire out. It would just crawl sideways past us and head up the hill. But it was spring and moisture had the advantage. After an hour the fire mostly burned itself out. Janette and I were exhausted.

There never was much threat to the cattle on top of the hill. We realized it. We downed the rest of the Kool-Aid. We knew we were going to get a whipping. You can't cover up that much smoke smell. We were resting before we went home. We were both concocting lies but we knew they would never work. The smell of smoke was too much.

Oren Gray came riding into our camp. He had seen the smoke. "Smoking will lead to a bad end," he said. "Isn't this view of the river and springtime good enough for you?" he asked. "Did you have to ruin it with stolen cigarettes and conflagration?"

I quickly figured out what "conflagration" means. I did not know how he knew we were smoking stolen cigarettes, but he knew. He probably knew about the Shack as well.

"It was her fault," I said. "She brought the matches and cigarettes."

He bowed his head; his old shoulders sagged and he shook his head and sighed. Janette would not look at him. She was pouting and angry.

Oren Gray said, "Same reaction. Different Eden." He sat in his saddle awhile looking at us. The leather creaked once or twice. Then he spoke. "You two are bad for one another. Avoid one another. You cause problems together. Boy, don't never get yoked with an unequal.

"This is my land and you know my fence line. Stay off my land because I have riders of my own who will hunt you down if you trespass. The foxes are welcome on my land—but not you. Now git!"

We left. I do not recall the consequences, but the next week a buyer showed up on our doorstep, made an offer, and Dad sold the farm. We moved from Holliday Creek to a village called Evanston, Iowa, east of the Hills, east of my boyhood Eden. After that we moved to Fort Dodge.

About The Author

David finished 3rd Grade at Holliday Creek School in June 1952. He was enrolled in Butler School in Fort Dodge, IA that September and graduated from Fort Dodge High in 1960. He earned his B.S. degree from Drake University in 1966 in English. He taught English at East High in Des Moines (1966-1972) where he joined the American Federation of Teachers (AFL/CIO) and carried a union card the rest of his teaching career.

David Wright married Polly Kaderabek in 1968 and their first daughter Wendy was born a year later. He earned an M.A. from Drake in 1972. That same year he secured a teaching position at Coronado High in Scottsdale, AZ. Their second daughter Sarah was born in 1974.

During his later years at Coronado, there was a strong trend to bring "curriculum integration" to the classroom. David Wright gained professional notoriety with his innovative program called Livengood. He promoted his ideas appearing frequently as a "break out speaker" at various teacher Conferences. He was contacted by the National Association of Secondary School Principals who requested that he explain his ideas about curriculum integration more fully. The result was Livengood: A Community Simulation Approach to

Integrative Education that appeared in their newsletter in January 1997. The NASSP article demonstrated how the disciplines of English, economics, math, are unified in a single program. The article showed how student empowerment and role playing work together in a project-driven curriculum. His article appeared again in Education Digest, March 1997. The program also earned a large grant from INTEL Corp. in a competition for innovative contributions to education. Curriculum Integration almost caught on in America, but the same tide that swept No Child Left Behind into power also swept curriculum integration out the door. After he retired from Scottsdale, David Wright re-entered the classroom teaching at the charter school Academy With Community Partners (2001-2008) in Mesa, Arizona. He still had a need to teach. Health problems forced his retirement in 2008. He has recovered since then and enjoys his family, travel and lots of golf. He and Polly spend quality time in the summer below the Mogollon Rim at Christopher Creek. A creek runs through it.

www.ingramcontent.com/pod-product-compliance
Lightning Source LLC
Chambersburg PA
CBHW051414280526
45785CB00003B/1064